RUN
WELL

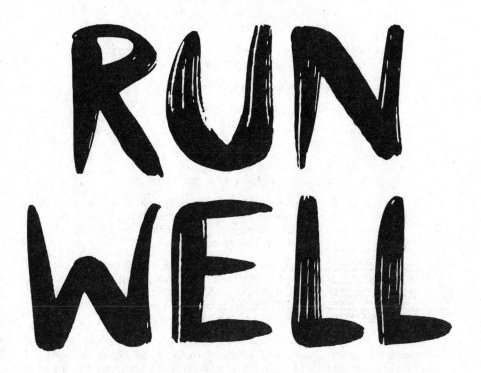

RUN WELL

Essential health questions and answers for runners

DR JULIET McGRATTAN

BLOOMSBURY SPORT
LONDON · OXFORD · NEW YORK · NEW DELHI · SYDNEY

BLOOMSBURY SPORT
Bloomsbury Publishing Plc
50 Bedford Square, London, WC1B 3DP, UK
29 Earlsfort Terrace, Dublin 2, Ireland

BLOOMSBURY, BLOOMSBURY SPORT and the Diana logo are trademarks
of Bloomsbury Publishing Plc

First published in Great Britain 2021

A catalogue record for this book is available from the British Library

Library of Congress Cataloguing-in-Publication data has been applied for

ISBN: TPB: 978-1-4729-7967-4; eBook: 978-1-4729-7964-3

2 4 6 8 10 9 7 5 3 1

Typeset in Source Serif by Deanta Global Publishing Services, Chennai, India
Printed and bound in Great Britain by CPI Group (UK) Ltd., Croydon, CR0 4YY

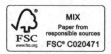

MIX
Paper from
responsible sources
FSC® C020471

To find out more about our authors and books visit www.bloomsbury.com
and sign up for our newsletters

CONTENTS

Preface *vii*

Introduction *1*

CHAPTER 1 The Head *3*

CHAPTER 2 The Cardiovascular System *28*

CHAPTER 3 The Respiratory System *49*

CHAPTER 4 The Gastrointestinal System *66*

CHAPTER 5 The Urinary System *87*

CHAPTER 6 The Reproductive System *109*

CHAPTER 7 The Musculoskeletal System *133*

CHAPTER 8 The Skin *172*

CHAPTER 9 Self-Care *200*

Acknowledgements *231*

References *233*

Index *244*

PREFACE

Dear Runner,

I have been a part of this wonderful community for 13 years and it has brought me so much joy. It has supported, encouraged and motivated me, helped me be my best, finished in front, behind and beside me, and cheered me on regardless. It's not just the running, it's the people and the opportunities that it has brought me. I have made friends, travelled the world and even found a new career. It was time for me to give back. I wanted to use my years of running, my 16 years working as a GP and my new career as a writer to create something for you all.

The human body is a complex and fascinating thing, and I am still learning about it. Despite our best intentions, things go wrong and navigating the online forums and websites to get the information you need can be a tricky and even dangerous task. Over the years as a GP and as a health expert for many magazines and online communities, I have been asked literally hundreds of running-related health questions. I hope in the pages of this book you will find something to reassure you, to inform you and even to make you laugh. I want you to learn about your body so you can be amazed by it, know how to look after it and feel confident about when to ask for help.

I have enjoyed writing this book so much. I have imagined you all, across the desk from my computer, asking me questions and listening to my answers. I feel you have shared this journey with me. So, my running friends, here is my book and I hope it helps you to run well.

P.S. Do remember that this book in no way replaces seeing a medical professional who can assess you, examine you and take your personal medical and family history into account. If you're a competing athlete, then always check that any medications you use aren't prohibited. But I know you know that!

INTRODUCTION

Running is a journey of discovery. Not just of running routes and new places but of your own human body. Your capacity to endure and perform. Your resilience and courage. Your ability to harness the power of running and use it in other areas of your life. But, like any journey, there are ups and downs, delays and set-backs. It's a steep learning curve with huge potential for errors but incredible rewards too.

I cast my mind back to my first half marathon. The New Balance English Half Marathon in Warrington in 2010. I had been running for two years and had never run more than 10 miles. I lined up at the start, already soaked and frozen from the torrential rain. I had no bin liner to keep me dry, no jumper to toss aside once I'd begun to run. I set off with no watch, no race fuel and wearing shorts that were not remotely designed for long distance running when you don't possess a thigh gap! It was the hardest thing I had ever done. My Dad was watching runner after runner cross the finish line and wondering if I had got lost. When I eventually did (just about) manage to raise my arms in celebration and claim my medal, I was broken. I could barely take another step or string a sentence together. My Dad bundled me into a restaurant, fed me pasta and drove me home. The next day I had such severe chafing that I had weeping wounds on my inner thighs. I had to use surgical dressings with tights over the top to even be able to walk. I couldn't wear a bra because the skin around my chest was so raw. My feet were one big blister. Everything hurt. Stairs were an impossibility, in fact, even turning over in bed made me wince and groan. I was a mess. But I was happy. I did it! I rose to what was a seemingly impossible challenge for me. I wanted more. I wanted to do it again and do it better, faster and with food, Vaseline and Lycra shorts! I knew I had a lot to learn about my body and myself. I was thirsty to find out the answers to all the questions I had.

That was the beginning of a true voyage of discovery for me. I want to share it with you. In this book I want to take you on a journey too, around your body. We'll visit each body system in turn, starting at the head and working our way down. We'll explore the anatomy and how each system works before turning to the questions that runners have asked me over the years. There'll be surprising facts, things to try at home and runners sharing their own experiences along our route. Grab your running shoes and water bottle. The starting gun has fired and the first stop is the brain.

CHAPTER 1

....

THE HEAD

F irmly protected inside our skull bones lies the control centre for our entire body. From regulating our breathing to determining our emotions, from activating muscles to weighing up facts, our brain masterminds it all. Despite extensive research we still don't fully understand how it works. Have you ever wondered whether running can make you more intelligent or why people get a headache after a run? And what exactly are the links between running and mental health? Let's get our heads down and explore this mind-blowingly clever part of our body.

The cerebral cortex is the outer part of the brain. It looks rather like a large, lumpy walnut and it's made up of four lobes: the frontal, parietal, temporal and occipital lobes. Each of these is responsible for different behaviours and functions.

The Brain

Frontal lobe: thinking, memory, behaviour, movement, decision making, planning and attention

Parietal lobe: language, touch, pain and taste

Temporal lobe: hearing, learning, feelings, speech, memory processing, emotions

Cerebellum: balance, co-ordination and posture

Brain stem: breathing, heart rate and temperature

Deeper inside the brain you'll find the midbrain, pons and medulla, which make up the brain stem. This controls a number of automatic functions, such as breathing, our heart rate and blood pressure. Behind the brain stem is the cerebellum, which is vital to us as runners, because it helps to control posture, balance and co-ordination. Other smaller areas of the brain include the thalamus, the hypothalamus, the limbic system and the basal ganglia. They all work closely together to make us who we are.

Brain cells are specialised cells called neurons and there are said to be nearly 100 billion of them in the brain. Neurons use chemical messages (neurotransmitters) and electrical impulses to communicate information around the brain and to the rest of the body at an astonishing speed. In return, neurons bring messages back to the brain, which processes them, takes into account other feedback from multiple sources, including glands which send their messages in the form of hormones, puts all the data together and determines what happens next. It's mind-boggling.

When you understand the functions of the different parts of the brain, it's easy to see how damage to one area can affect particular body functions or behaviours. Medical research is still trying to unpick exactly what goes on inside the brain and how exercise can influence it, but let's look at some of the knowledge we have so far and answer some questions. We'll then move on to look at headaches, eyes and ears, all of which can pose important issues in the heads of runners.

Q I know running improves my mental health, but how?

A Running is a very powerful tool for keeping you mentally well. First, we know that running causes chemical changes in the brain, releasing endorphins – substances that make you feel good both during and for a time after a run. Alongside this, running and other types of exercise also have an anti-inflammatory effect in the body. We know that many major diseases, including depression, are partly caused by a long-term, low-grade inflammation. This inflammation is caused by a number of factors, but one of them is inactivity. Running can help to counteract this, because it not only reduces harmful internal fat in the body (a significant cause of inflammation), but also causes the muscles to release anti-inflammatory proteins called myokines.

Aside from the chemistry of physical exercise, running can help you develop a positive sense of self. Setting targets and reaching goals can help build self-esteem and confidence. It can make you appreciate the power that your body has and what it can actually achieve, which is usually way beyond what you thought your capabilities were. Running also brings people into your life. We know that having a sense of belonging and feeling part of a community is important for mental wellbeing. Whether that is a virtual community online, one running buddy to share your journey with or a whole parkrun family, that sense of knowing that others champion and support you, and that you can contribute to other peoples' lives in a positive way, is very rewarding and fulfilling. This sense of belonging also extends to places as well as people. If you're running outside and off the treadmill then running connects you with nature, which has a calming effect, encourages us to feel gratitude and brings wellbeing.

Did you know?

Any exercise can improve mood, stress and anxiety, but exercising in green spaces outdoors has been shown to have a greater calming effect than exercising indoors. Researchers looking at data from the Scottish Health Survey in 2008 found that exercising in parks or woodland was 50 per cent better for mental wellbeing than exercising in a gym. It's not yet fully understood why and how the brain responses vary in different environments.

Q What is a runner's high?

When you run, the body releases endorphins, which are feel-good chemicals that give you a sense of wellbeing. Endorphins bind to the same receptors in the brain as opiates such as morphine do, making you feel relaxed and happy. A runner's high is much more than this, though. It's a euphoric sensation. When you run long distances you can feel completely invincible, all pain disappears and you are literally on top of the world with no sense of time. Strangely it doesn't happen consistently, so it's not just a case of running, getting a few endorphins into your bloodstream and having a high. Many runners have never experienced a true runner's high. Have you?

I have, but only twice, and despite running many marathons since, I haven't been able to reproduce that intense feeling of ecstasy while out running.

Researchers have been trying to solve this conundrum, which is a tricky one, because a runner's high is a very personal experience and is difficult to measure. They suspect that it is far more complicated than just the release of endorphins. Evidence is pointing to the involvement of endocannabinoids – cannabis-like chemicals produced by the body and released during exercise. High levels of endocannabinoids have been found in the blood of endurance athletes and the characteristic sensations of pain relief, psychological changes and the easing of anxiety that can occur with cannabis plant use mirror that of a runner's high. It's interesting that the same euphoric episodes don't seem to happen in other sports and there's something about the experience of endurance running that invokes this state. Perhaps it's yet another indicator that we were born to run and without our need to chase and hunt our prey we instead chase and reach for the often-elusive runner's high.

Q Can you get addicted to running?

 Addiction is the inability to stop consuming a substance or taking part in an activity even though it's causing you psychological or physical harm. It may be a substance addiction such as alcohol or a behavioural addiction such as gambling. What starts as a voluntary activity that you choose to do becomes one that you can't control and are dependent on to cope with everyday life.

There's no doubt that running makes you feel good and creates the urge to go out and do it again – it's enjoyable! – but when you think about the runner's high and explore the possible role of opiate-like endorphins and endocannabinoids, it's easy to see how running could become an addictive behaviour. You can crave the way that running makes you feel and go out to get your fix. However, what is important here is whether it is causing you any harm and whether you have control over whether or not you run. Consider the following questions:

- Are you running despite having an injury and being advised not to?
- Are you obsessed and running yourself into the ground when you know you should rest?
- Is your running having a negative effect on your family, but, although you know this, you just can't stop?
- Has running become a compulsive behaviour, one that you can't control?
- Do you fear that something bad will happen if you don't run?
- Do you feel guilty or ashamed after you've run?
- What happens when you don't run – do you experience withdrawal symptoms?
- Are you choosing to run?

These are all questions to consider when deciding whether your relationship with running is a healthy one. It's very easy to say, 'I'm addicted to running,' but in reality, an addiction is a serious medical issue that needs expert help to overcome. You should always run because you choose to, not because you have to. Over-training can lead to health issues (see page 204), both physical and mental and it's important to find the right balance for you.

Q Will running improve my intelligence?

A There's no doubt that going for a run clears your head and makes it easier for you to sit down and focus afterwards, but can it actually make you smarter, improve your capacity for learning and increase your memory recall? It's a myth that we are born with a certain number of brain cells and as we age they gradually die off. Yes, we do lose brain cells (neurons), but new ones are made too, thousands every day, in a process called neurogenesis. It's important to know that much of the research in this area has been carried out on rats and extrapolated to humans, but numerous studies have shown that exercise stimulates neurogenesis in the hippocampus of laboratory animals, the part of the brain which is used for spatial memory. Spatial memory is our ability to orientate ourselves, find our way around a place and remember where we put things. We can't directly measure neuron numbers in a living human hippocampus, but studies looking at the blood flow in this part of the brain confirm that it significantly increases with exercise, suggesting new brain cell growth.

A study from Finland found that rats that ran the furthest had the largest number of neurons in the hippocampus. Short, high intensity exercise and resistance training (such as lifting weights) had little or no effect, so endurance running may have a special ability to improve spatial memory. I read an interesting piece highlighting that this might be an evolutionary function, because our descendants often had to run many miles to chase down prey and a superior ability to know where they were and how to get home was a survival essential!

The brain protein called brain-derived neurotrophic factor (BDNF) helps promote neurogenesis and it's now thought that another protein called cathepsin B (CTSB), a myokine secreted by muscles, has a role to play too. Its secretion is activated by exercise and in a study done on humans, people who exercised consistently, performed better in memory tests and had higher CTSB levels in the blood.

Interestingly, it's thought that while exercise might increase the number of neurons, if they aren't used those cells can quickly die. Brain training can help retain them, so a combination of exercise and simultaneous brain training produces the biggest and most enduring increase in neurogenesis. Try challenging yourself to learn a tricky running drill or cross-train by mastering a dance routine – it might be the ideal way to hold onto those new brain cells. It seems that running doesn't necessarily make you smarter, but it can produce the new brain cells that put you in the best state for learning.

Did you know?

A 2014 study by Stanford University found that people are 60 per cent more creative when they're walking. It was the movement itself rather than the environment which made the difference, so grabbing some exercise in your lunch break, even if it's through uninspiring city streets, could fill you with ideas for an afternoon meeting.

Q Will running reduce my risk of dementia?

As we age, our cognitive functions – in other words our ability to learn and understand, including processes such as memory, thinking and problem-solving – generally decline. The good news is that research has shown that exercising regularly will help to maintain our cognitive functions. In 2011, a meta-analysis of studies showed that in people who don't have dementia, exercise helped to stop cognitive decline. Those who exercised the most had the greatest protection (38 per cent), but those who exercised at low or moderate levels still benefited significantly (35 per cent), so any exercise is good.

Dementia is characterised by progressive memory loss and although it tends to happen over the age of 65 (any earlier than this and it is referred to as early onset dementia), dementia is not simply a consequence of natural ageing, it is a medical condition. The different types of dementia affect the brain in different ways, for example, in Alzheimer's disease, protein plaques develop in the brain, which gradually affect its function. In vascular dementia, a lack of blood flow to different areas of the brain causes damage to the brain tissue. Dementia is a medical condition and is not inevitable.

So can running help to prevent us getting dementia? Some cases of dementia are inherited, particularly the young-onset cases, but generally the news is good. Exercise on its own has been shown to reduce the risk of dementia by up to six per cent. If, however, you combine that with other lifestyle measures such as lowering your blood pressure, not smoking and maintaining a normal weight, then the reduction may be as high as 40 per cent, particularly in the case of vascular dementia. It's important to remember too that regular exercise is vital in the care of those who already have dementia, as it can help maintain independence, give a better quality of life and boost self-esteem.

Did you know?

Dementia UK reports there are over 200 subtypes of dementia. Alzheimer's disease is the most common type in the UK followed by vascular dementia. Other types include dementia with Lewy bodies, frontotemporal dementia and mixed dementia.

Q I love running, but have a really busy life. If I run, I just spend the whole time thinking and worrying about all the other things I should be doing.

A When life is chaotic and each day is crammed with a long list of 'to dos', then it's easy to either not run at all or not enjoy your run. First of all, you must lose any guilt you have about running. It's not selfish or indulgent to take a bit of time for yourself to exercise. In fact, it is essential for you as a busy person. You will be far better equipped to deal with all life throws at you if you use exercise to keep you physically and mentally well. YOU need to be at the top of your priority list. Always make sure your to-do list is realistic. There's nothing more disheartening than getting to the end of every day with a long list of things you haven't done. Only schedule in what you think you can manage and move the rest to another day.

Have a look at your time management. There are only ever going to be 24 hours in a day and it's often how cleverly we spend them that determines how much we get through. Check for activities that drain your time, such as scrolling through social media. It's easy to reduce this by the half an hour needed for a run. Look for life hacks that will free up time and see what you can delegate to family or friends. You simply can't do everything!

When you are actually running, there are a couple of things you can try to stop you worrying. Both mindful running and productive running can help. Learning to calm your mind and focus on the present will really help you to relax and enjoy your run. Similarly, using a run to solve a specific problem is a great use of precious time. The boxes below have techniques that can transform your running, so I urge you to give them a try.

Mindful running

TRY THIS AT HOME

If you're one of those people who is always distracted when you're running, thinking about what you need to do when you get back from your run and not taking the time to enjoy the run itself, then try mindful running. Being able to focus on that exact moment in time will calm your busy mind and help you get the most out of your run for *you*. Here is my favourite way to stay present using the senses:

- Take a few minutes before you run to sit or stand quietly and take some deep belly breaths (see page 59). As you breathe out, feel the tension leaving your body. Don't skip this step – you can't go straight from rushing about to mindful running.
- Don't run distracted. Don't set a goal pace or interval session. Ideally leave your sports watch and your headphones at home.
- When you run, think about what you can feel. Notice your breathing and try to keep it calm. Feel the beat of your heart in your chest. Feel the air as it brushes your skin. Feel the sensation as your feet hit the ground. Are your shoulders tense? Try to relax them. Do you feel strong? It's OK if you feel tired, just acknowledge it.

continued overleaf ▶

- When you run, think about what you can hear. The repetitive thud of your feet on the ground. The birds. The wind. The traffic. Children playing. Take time to notice each sound.
- When you run, think about what you can see. Take in your surroundings. The light and shadows. The sky. The shapes of trees and buildings. Like a child, notice the small things. The ladybird on the leaf. The colours on the road sign. Open your eyes – we miss so much when we run.
- When you run, think about what you can taste. The mint of your toothpaste. The sweetness of a sports drink. The salty sea air.
- When you run, think about what you can smell. Freshly cut grass. The fumes from the lorry that passes. Garlic wafting from the Italian restaurant. Pleasant or unpleasant, notice the smells.
- Try one of the above or spend a little time on each during your run. It will keep your mind focused and enjoying the present rather than ruminating on the past or worrying about the future.
- Take a few minutes at the end of your run to take some deep, gentle breaths again. Feel how calm you are. Try to carry on with your day in this relaxed state.

Productive running

TRY THIS AT HOME

Productive running is a great tool, particularly for those that are time-pressured. Running has as amazing ability to help us solve problems and great ideas often spring to mind during a run. Productive running is all about harnessing these benefits. Try this technique and I promise you'll be impressed by the result:

- Choose something difficult you need to achieve such as creating a presentation for work, figuring out how to deal with a tricky situation or writing a challenging letter.
- Choose a route that doesn't involve lots of road crossings or technical running so your mind is free.

continued overleaf ▶

- While you're putting on your trainers or during your warm-up, set your intention for what you want to achieve during the run. Think about how good you'll feel coming home with this task done.
- When you're running try to keep your mind on the topic. One of the joys of running is being able to let your mind wander, but for productive running you need to keep focused on the problem.
- When your thoughts stray from the task, gently guide them back to the problem. If you have ever meditated, you'll know how often this wandering happens when you first start. It gets easier with practice.
- Work through your task, step by step. Don't keep going over and over the bit you have already solved (trust me, it's very tempting), keep moving forwards. Depending on the challenge, you might need a longer or a shorter run.
- As soon as your run is over, write down anything that you need to remember – it's amazing how quickly things can vanish from your mind! Alternatively, use the voice recorder on your phone to make a note while you're running along.

With this technique you can turn a run into a productive time where you'll be able to focus, concentrate and be very creative. Give it a try next time you need to solve a problem. I don't suggest you do this with every run, though, as the benefits from mind-wandering runs are very important too!

Q I really struggle with finding the motivation to run, even though I know I'll feel good afterwards.

A This is really normal, so don't worry. As running legend Kathrine Switzer said, 'The hardest part of any workout is putting your shoes on.' There aren't many runners who always feel like running and just getting out the door can be a huge challenge to all of us. Here are some things that might help:

- **Run with others** Enlist the help of running friends. Knowing someone is expecting you will make you go. Think about joining a running club – not only will there be club sessions to commit to, but you'll meet other runners who will always be happy to help keep you motivated.
- **Run commute** Make running a normal part of your day. Whether it's running home from work or on the way back from the school drop-off, if you have a set time and routine that you follow, then habits are easier to establish.
- **Just run for 10 minutes** Just tell yourself you'll go out and see how you feel. You can come home if you want to, but I can almost guarantee that once you've been out running for 10 minutes you'll feel as if you might as well carry on for a bit longer.
- **Schedule your runs** Planning is key. Look at the week ahead, decide when you could run and then add it to your calendar. It's an appointment with yourself and it must only be changed in an emergency, because your health is high priority. This stops you getting to the end of a busy week and suddenly realising you haven't fitted in a run.
- **Don't over think it** Procrastination is fatal. It's so easy to talk yourself out of a run or spend so long thinking about it that you miss your window of opportunity. Just run. You might find that the morning is best, and you can lay your clothes out the night before, so you're up and out before engaging your brain. Similarly, run before you come home from work or you'll just end up getting in and putting the kettle on. Don't over think it.
- **Find inspiration** Watching a marathon on television will stir the desire to run in even the most unmotivated of people, so fill your life with inspiration. It might be your own running diary that reminds you how good running makes you feel, books, podcasts, TV documentaries or online running forums. Whatever it is, a regular dose can keep you fired up.

- **Volunteer** Go and volunteer at your local parkrun or marshal at a local event. You'll be welcomed with open arms, and watching others run and chatting to them afterwards will get you back on track. You'll also feel proud to be involved with the running community in a different way.

If your lack of motivation is persistent and associated with a low mood or feelings of self-doubt or hopelessness, then it's time to reach out for some help. These can all be symptoms of depression, so make an appointment to discuss it with your doctor.

DEPRESSION AND ANXIETY

Q I think I'm depressed, but don't want to take antidepressants. I know running helps depression, but will it be enough?

A Exercise has been shown to be more effective than doing nothing when it comes to reducing the symptoms of depression. Some studies have shown it to be as effective as certain antidepressants. Exercise is never the wrong thing to do in this situation, but take care if you are already running regularly and have become depressed. Just keeping on running or running more is unlikely to be the answer, although stopping running will almost certainly have a negative effect. It can, however, be really hard to motivate yourself to run when your mood is low and even simple everyday tasks are a struggle. If going for a run feels impossible or too overwhelming, then it's equally OK not to go. You can get better without running and it doesn't solve everything.

It would be really good to talk it all through with someone and your GP would be an ideal person. They will be able to help you assess how severely affected you are and whether lifestyle changes are enough. Sometimes the act of simply talking and admitting there is a problem can be therapeutic and there is no need to struggle alone. You may not want antidepressants, but there are also talking therapies and counselling that you may benefit from. Your GP will be able to refer you. If you and your doctor come to a decision together that using an antidepressant is the right step for you, then it's important not to see this as a failure. It can be a very effective treatment and is life-changing for many. There's even some evidence that regular exercise can help to enhance the effects of some antidepressants, so don't stop running, but do seek help and support.

Real-life runners

Running and being outdoors has always left me with a fresh perspective and the potential for new opportunities. I think being free, without distractions, is an occasion not to be missed, and will pay dividends to your mental fitness.

Louise Goddard, LegItLancaster running community

Q If I run regularly can I stop my antidepressants?

A You should never stop your antidepressants without speaking to your doctor. There are two main reasons for this. First, you may need a gradual withdrawal from your medication, depending on which one you are taking. Coming off antidepressants can sometimes be difficult and can take time, so it needs to be approached in the right way. Second, it's easy to get carried away when you first feel better and end up stopping your medication too early. You may then get a relapse in your low mood, which can be very upsetting as you thought you were feeling OK. It's good to have a period of a few months when you feel well and stable before you look at stopping antidepressants. It's best to make this decision in conjunction with your doctor and a friend or family member. It can help to make a list of the symptoms and behaviours that you experienced when you first realised you were depressed, so that you and your nominated person can watch out for them. For example, did you become anti-social, lose your appetite or begin to have difficulty sleeping? If a pattern emerges it enables you to take prompt action and seek support.

Regular exercise, such as running, is a really important part of treatment for depression. It can be a vital tool for keeping you well, both when you're on medication and after you stop taking it. Having running as a coping mechanism will help you to deal with life events and maintain good mental health. Positive lifestyle changes, such as increasing your exercise, may also speed up your recovery time and prevent relapses, but despite this there are many people who still need their antidepressants regularly.

Did you know?

The World Health Organisation states that one in four people in the world will be affected by a mental disorder at some point during their lives. It's one of the leading causes of ill health and disability worldwide. The mental health charity Mind tells us that, in England, in any given week, one in six of us will experience a mental health problem including depression and anxiety. It's OK not to be OK.

Q I feel anxious about going outside. Will running help?

A In the same way that the chemical changes in the brain induced by running can improve mood, they can also have a calming effect, which can ease symptoms of anxiety. Having anxiety makes you hyperalert, jittery and very often afraid. With your heart racing and breathing rate increased, your body is ready to fight a threat, even when no real threat exists – and it can be mentally and physically exhausting. Anxiety can come in sudden and short-lived attacks, either out of the blue or in response to a particular trigger, or it can be a more generalised anxiety with a constant feeling of worry and self-doubt. Whatever the type of anxiety, it can lead to a fear of leaving the house as remaining within the confines of your own four walls feels safer. Getting out for a run, though, will help you. Your breathing will calm and the racing thoughts in your head will settle down (see page 5). You'll experience the fresh air and nurturing benefits of nature, and if you struggle with fitful sleep it will help that too (see page 220). You'll also feel proud that you made it out of the door and achieved something, which will give you a positive feedback loop and spur you on to do it again.

It can be easier said than done, though, so be gentle with yourself. It's better to set and achieve a realistic target than to overestimate, put too much pressure on yourself and fail. To begin with, running 50 metres up the road and back might be enough. Consider asking someone for help. Having the reassurance of a friend running with you or cycling alongside you can make all the difference. Not only can it give you the motivation and confidence to get out of the door in the first place, but it also provides the opportunity to chat, which can distract you from your anxiety. It's also much easier to open up and share your feelings when you're side by side and not face to face.

Real-life runners

Running has transformed my health and wellbeing both physically and mentally. It's helped me cope with the death of my dad. My dad's brother died just after him and at the second funeral in two weeks I saw one of my cousins, Kevin, who is named after my dad. I asked him what he was doing tomorrow. He said, 'I'm running the Dublin marathon. You should do it one day.' I agreed and my running journey began. The rest is history.

Mike Whelan, runner and Leinster Rugby fanatic

EARS

Q I suddenly felt dizzy on my last run and had to walk home. What could have caused that?

A So many things cause dizziness. Doctors often need to do a bit of detective work and ask questions about a whole range of body systems to figure out the reason it's happening and, even then, the cause might remain unknown. Feeling a bit light-headed can come from simply over exerting yourself or being a little dehydrated or hungry. Feeling anxious can make you dizzy too. Dizziness associated with other symptoms, such as palpitations or chest pain, can be due to anaemia, a drop in blood pressure or more serious heart conditions (see page 34). Similarly, dizziness with an accompanying shortness of breath or cough can result from both minor or major lung conditions. Dizziness with double vision and numbness or weakness could be a migraine or, at its worst, a stroke. Thankfully most dizziness isn't serious and settles on its own.

One source of dizziness is the ear. Ears not only deliver hearing, but also control balance. There's a network of tunnels in each ear called the semi-circular canals, which are lined with tiny hairs and filled with fluid. When you move your head, the fluid moves. This causes the hairs to move and messages are then sent to your brain, which interprets your position. Anything which disrupts the movement of the hairs will result in incorrect or abnormal messages being sent. An infection of the inner ear, such as a viral labyrinthitis or small crystals, called otoconia, floating in the canal, can disrupt the fluid movement. Rather than simply feeling dizzy, with these conditions you might experience vertigo, where things around you appear to spin.

The important factors with dizziness are whether it is a one-off or a recurrent problem; whether it is short-lived or long-lasting; and what the associated symptoms are. Dizziness usually goes away on its own and if you feel dizzy it's always best to lie down and drink plenty of fluid. Take care to get up slowly when you feel better. For anything other than a short spell of dizziness with an obvious cause, it's best to discuss it with your doctor who may recommend medication or arrange investigations to determine the cause.

Q I keep getting itching and infections just inside my ear. Could running be to blame?

A You might have heard of swimmer's ear, also known as otitis externa. Inflammation or infection develops in the skin of the ear canal, which leads from the outside to the ear drum. The canal gets itchy, sore and can become sticky with a discharge. It's called swimmer's ear, because it occurs most often in people whose ears are frequently wet. If you're someone who always runs in the rain or frequently showers, then you might be at more risk of developing it, but the biggest risk is for runners who spend hours with ear buds in. The ear buds trap moisture inside the ear, which can irritate the skin and provide a perfect environment for germs to grow. To avoid the problem, don't wear ear buds for an excessive amount of time and take care to dry your ears after they've been wet. Simply wipe around the outside part with the corner of a clean towel or tissue or waft warm air from a hair dryer into your ear, but don't use a cotton bud to dry inside the canal. Make sure you keep your ear buds clean too. Otitis externa can be treated with ear drops from the pharmacy, but an established infection may need treatment from your doctor.

EYES

Q Why do my eyes water when I run?

A It can be so frustrating when each time you run you have tears streaming down your face. Eye irritation while running is common and can lead to blurred vision (see question below) and general annoyance. Tears are one of the many ways our body protects itself. They lubricate and stop the surface of the eye from drying out, and prevent foreign bodies, such as dust, getting into the eye, but sometimes they seem to work overtime. Tears are made in the lacrimal glands situated at the top of the eye and they drain away through the tear ducts. You can see a tiny hole leading to the tear duct in the inner corner of your upper and lower lids if you look closely. Tear production might increase if your eye is drying out in cold, hot or windy weather. Eyes might also stream if they are irritated by pollen, dust or fumes. Sometimes people with dry eyes find that their eyes water a lot, which might sound strange, but it's just the eye trying to correct the dryness. If you're affected, try to work out what your trigger is. If it's pollen, then an antihistamine eye drop might do the trick.

Sunglasses will help to keep pollen out, and can also stop dust and bright light affecting your eyes. If you generally have dry eyes, then you can buy a simple lubricating eye drop from the pharmacy to use regularly and before you run. If your eyes water all the time, not just when you run, then it might be due to an infection or a blocked tear duct stopping the tears from draining away, so see your doctor if it persists.

Q I got blurry vision on my last long run. Should I be worried?

A Eyes are so precious and it's advisable to get advice about any new or unexplained eye problem. Vision can become blurred for a number of minor and some more major reasons too, so be cautious. Minor reasons include irritation of the cornea (surface), which can dry out quickly in the cold and wind (this is a particular problem for contact lens wearers). Sun cream or sweat running into the eyes can also cause irritation. If something flies into your eye and scratches the cornea, even if it flies out again, it can cause some discomfort and altered vision. This is called a corneal abrasion and while our eye lashes and tears are designed to protect our eyes, sometimes the unexpected happens on a run, particularly on a breezy day. Excess tears in the eyes can cause blurred vision too.

If your blood pressure is unusually low and making you feeling faint, then you might have less blood flowing to the part of your brain which controls vision and may experience some blurring as a result. People often cite low blood sugar as a possible cause of blurred vision, but this is unusual unless you are a diabetic on medication that puts you at risk of hypoglycaemic (low blood sugar) attacks. Blurred vision, an area of darkness or some zig-zag lines in your field of vision are typical symptoms of a migraine aura. It may or may not develop into a full-blown migraine.

While all these causes are reversible and unlikely to cause permanent damage, it's important to know that blurred vision can be a sign of something more sinister. If it's associated with floaters (black specs floating around like dust in front of your eyes), flashes of light or a curtain appearing to block off some of your visual field, then this is potentially a detachment of your retina and you need to seek an urgent medical assessment as this can cause permanent damage to your vision. Similarly, a stroke that affects your eye can present with a change in vision in one eye. It can become double or blurred or you may lose sight completely. If a stroke affects the visual centre in the brain, then it may cause these changes in both eyes simultaneously. You may or may not have other symptoms of a stroke.

A rarer cause is a condition called optic neuritis where the optic nerve, which carries information between the eyes and the brain, becomes inflamed. If you have optic neuritis it may become apparent after a run, with reduced, blurred vision and pain in the eye, especially when you try to move it in different directions. Optic neuritis needs to be diagnosed and investigated by a specialist to ensure no other medical conditions, such as multiple sclerosis, underlie it.

Blurred vision that develops slowly over time can have many other causes that aren't directly related to running. Don't try to self-diagnose. If you have new visual changes then get assessed. If you suspect a stroke or a detached retina, then these are medical emergencies and you should go to Accident and Emergency. If you have a mild or recurrent problem, then see your optician or GP.

Q Exercise seems to be good at preventing so many diseases. Does it help prevent eye disease too?

A Reading about blurred vision above you might feel a little worried that exercise is bad for your eyes, but in fact it's quite the opposite! Exercising regularly can help protect your eye health. Many serious eye diseases are linked to high blood pressure, high cholesterol and diabetes, which exercise is well known to help either prevent or manage. Take glaucoma, for example, a leading cause of blindness worldwide, where pressure builds up inside the eye. Some studies have shown that exercise may lower the pressure inside the eye. One study done in 2017 found that moderate to vigorous exercise might be particularly beneficial. The participants who were the most physically active had a 73 per cent lower incidence of glaucoma than the least active. For every 10-minute increase in this type of physical activity per week, the risk of glaucoma decreased by 25 per cent. If you already have glaucoma, then vigorous exercise may not be suitable for you, so please check with your ophthalmologist. Similarly, several studies found that people who exercised were less likely to develop a common eye condition called age-related macular degeneration (AMD) than those who were sedentary and didn't exercise. The macular is part of the retina at the back of the eye. When it degenerates central vision is lost and the periphery is spared, so although you don't lose your vision completely it can be very debilitating. There is still much we don't understand about the link between the two, but it seems clear that we can add eye health to our list of reasons why we run.

HEADACHES

Q Why do I get a headache after I run?

A Safety first. If you get a severe, sudden onset of a headache during a high intensity workout, where you feel as if someone has hit you over the back of the head, then this is a medical emergency. This could be a burst blood vessel in the brain causing a subarachnoid haemorrhage (SAH), where blood bleeds onto the surface of the brain. SAH is more common over the age of 50 and happens when small swellings on blood vessels, called aneurysms, burst. The severe headache may be associated with vomiting, double vision or even a loss of consciousness. It is a type of stroke so you should dial 999 for an emergency ambulance.

What is much more common, however, is a headache which starts when you come back from a run or even later that day. There are lots of reasons why this can happen and thankfully most of them are reversible, so you should be able to avoid a post-run headache:

- **Dehydration** You can lose lots of body water when you run, through your breath as well as your sweat, so make sure you adequately replace your losses, because dehydration is a major cause of headache. This might mean drinking extra fluid in the hours after you run, rather than just relying on a quick post-run guzzle.

- **Hunger** If you haven't properly fuelled your run, then a headache might strike. People don't often feel hungry straight after a long run, but if you frequently get a headache, then eating within half an hour of stopping might prevent it.
- **Poor running posture** Carrying tension in your neck and shoulders can trigger headaches. Try to relax your shoulders, holding them down and back, and keeping your head held high. You might benefit from intermittently shaking your arms out and circling your shoulders.
- **The weather** A blast of cold air to the head or a strong wind can bring on a headache. Some people find air pressure is a trigger and tend to get headaches on heavy, muggy days. We can't change the weather, but we can wear hats, cover our ears with headbands and take a paracetamol if we're badly affected.
- **Bright sunlight** Headaches often strike on very bright sunny days when the sun's glare is strong. Many runners say they don't like running in sunglasses, but if you invest in a lightweight pair that fits you well then you won't even notice they're there. Wraparound glasses will really keep the light out and a hat with a brim will help too.

Q Will running improve my migraines?

A This very much depends on what causes your migraines. Sometimes they happen out of the blue, but very often there's a trigger and this may be where running can help. For example, if sleep deprivation is a trigger for you, then it's reassuring to know that regular running can help you sleep (see page 220). Similarly, if stress is a frequent cause of your migraines then using running to help you manage your stress levels could be life-changing. Lots of the triggers such as diet, alcohol and hormonal changes can't be improved by running, but sometimes a gentle run will ease a mild headache from a migraine. It's important to be aware that running could potentially trigger migraines so make sure you know how to avoid post-run headaches.

TOP TIPS FOR A HEALTHY RUNNER'S HEAD

- Run regularly to get the most benefits from running.
- Find your tribe. A real or virtual community will support and motivate you.
- Head outside to run whenever you can to get the boost that nature gives your mood and brain power.
- Know that you are enough. You have nothing to prove.
- Be happy without running. Make sure that your happiness doesn't depend on running. You should be happy and fulfilled without it.
- Don't let running become a pressure. Check in with yourself intermittently to make sure you are enjoying your running.
- Volunteer regularly or from time to time. Giving back to others, including the running community, is rewarding and life-enriching.
- Never be afraid to ask for help. Find someone you trust to share your thoughts and problems with.

FURTHER HELP AND ADVICE

Mind: www.mind.org.uk
Moodcafe: www.moodcafe.co.uk
Anxiety UK: www.anxietyuk.org.uk
Action on Addiction: www.actiononaddiction.org.uk
The Samaritans: www.samaritans.org
Macular Society: www.macularsociety.org
International Glaucoma Association: www.glaucoma-association.com
The Migraine Trust: www.migrainetrust.org
Dementia UK: www.dementiauk.org
Headspace: www.headspace.com

CHAPTER 2

....

THE CARDIOVASCULAR SYSTEM

There is no denying that running is good for your heart. The heart is a muscle and by using it regularly, gradually increasing the work you ask it to do and looking after it, it will become stronger and more efficient. Regular running can reduce your risk of developing coronary heart disease and stroke by 30 per cent. From blood pressure to palpitations, from a family history of heart disease to freezing cold fingers, running and circulation questions are many and varied. This chapter explores them all and also gives you tips on how to keep your heart healthy.

The heart collects blood that has already made its journey around the body, pumps it to the lungs, where it is replenished with oxygen, and then forcefully pumps this oxygenated blood to the organs and muscles. A fast, continuous supply of oxygen-rich blood is essential for skeletal muscles to function and perform well during running. A good blood supply is also needed to take away the waste products that result from exercise.

The Circulatory System

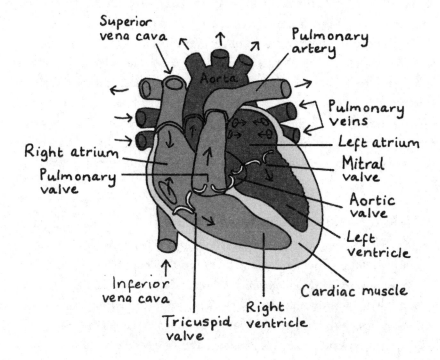

Superior vena cava

Aorta

Pulmonary artery

Pulmonary veins

Left atrium

Right atrium

Mitral valve

Pulmonary valve

Aortic valve

Left ventricle

Inferior vena cava

Cardiac muscle

Tricuspid valve

Right ventricle

The collecting chambers of the heart are called the atria and the pumping chambers are called the ventricles. There are valves between these to prevent blood flowing in the wrong direction. Large veins called the superior and inferior vena cava bring blood that has circulated around the body to the right atrium. The right atrium pumps it into the right ventricle, which then pumps it to the lungs via the pulmonary artery. Once it has been enriched with oxygen in the lungs, the blood returns to the heart via the pulmonary veins. It collects in the left atrium, which pumps it into the left ventricle. The left ventricle is the strongest pumping chamber as from there the blood exits via the aorta (the body's biggest artery) and makes its way around the entire body, giving up its oxygen to tissues and organs before returning back to the heart via the veins.

The average person has approximately 5 litres of blood in their body (women have slightly less than men). It takes about one minute for that entire volume to go once around the body and back to the heart. When you exercise, however, that increases by four to five times. So when you're pounding your way down that finishing straight, your heart could be pumping 20 to 25 litres per minute! That's an incredible amount and you can see why running is an intense workout for your heart.

Thankfully, the heart muscle, or cardiac muscle as it's known, responds well to training. As it strengthens, the force of the contractions and therefore the effectiveness of the pump increases, and more blood is pumped in one heartbeat. A heart that is used to working hard when you're running will find life pretty easy when you're at rest. This is why, as you get fitter, you will see a reduction in your resting heart rate. It's very satisfying to see this number falling as your fitness increases.

Resting heart rate

TRY THIS AT HOME

You can measure your resting heart rate by feeling your pulse first thing in the morning, before you get out of bed. Count how many times it beats in 30 seconds and then double it to calculate your pulse rate in beats per minute. Resting heart rate varies by age and gender, but an average would be 70 beats per minute. A fit runner could expect a resting heart rate of around 60 beats per minute, but some highly trained athletes can have a rate as low as 30 to 40 beats per minute. Keep a record of your resting heart rate and watch it fall as you get fitter. If it increases, it may be a sign that you are training too hard, have an illness or are suffering stress; consider an easier session or a rest day.

Did you know?

Heart rate variability (HRV) might help us to manage our wellbeing. HRV is a measure of the variation in time between our heart beats. It's controlled by our autonomic nervous system. When you're relaxed and well, the HRV is high. Low HRV has been linked to cardiovascular disease, depression and anxiety. Heart rate monitors and apps can help you track your HRV and you will see it increase as you become fitter and more relaxed.

Q What should my maximum heart rate be when I'm exercising?

A Due to technological advances in recording body stats and also because they want to use it for training purposes, more and more runners are measuring their heart rate. Generally, the harder you work and the more effort you put in, the faster your heart will go. The most accurate way to find out your maximum heart rate (MHR) is by being measured using specialised equipment while on a static bike or treadmill. Obviously, we don't all have access to this, so there are many equations for calculating what your MHR should be and one of the simplest is 220 minus your age. So, at age 45, your MHR should be about 175 beats per minute (220 minus 45). As you get older, your MHR decreases. However, your heart rate depends on factors other than age, including body size, medical conditions and how fit you are. No one size fits all – isn't that always the way?

As a general guide, exercise should be done at between 50 to 85 per cent of your MHR (88 to 149 for a 45-year-old). When you're training well below your MHR you'll be able to sustain running for longer periods of time. The closer you are to your MHR, the harder it will be to keep going. As you get fitter, you can push your heart rate closer to its maximum for longer and even increase your MHR.

Heart rate can be used to direct your training. Your long slow runs should be done at 50 to 70 per cent of your MHR, threshold and tempo runs at 70 to 85 per cent of MHR, and short intervals at above 85 per cent of MHR. You should spend time in all of these zones for good all-round training. It's all about setting the training zones that are right for you and adapting them as you get fitter. If you're interested in heart rate training – and it's not for everyone – then there are lots of useful resources online and you can consider working with a running coach experienced in the field.

Remember, though, that you can use your perceived effort, for example whether you're gasping for breath or can talk, to guide your training in the same way, without having to measure anything (see page 62).

Q I had my blood pressure measured at work and was told it's high and I need to see my doctor. Can I carry on running?

A The medical term for high blood pressure is hypertension, and regular exercise is crucial in preventing and treating it. Whether it's safe for you to run right now depends on how high your blood pressure (BP) is.

A BP measurement is made up of two numbers, for example 120/70. The first number is called the systolic value and reflects the maximum pressure in your circulatory system when your heart is beating. The second number is the diastolic value and represents the lowest pressure when your heart is resting between beats. Blood pressure is measured in mmHg (millimetres of mercury), even though mercury is no longer used in blood pressure machines. When you see your doctor or nurse, if your BP is 140/90 or above, then you will need further tests to confirm the diagnosis of hypertension. The NICE guidelines from 2019 advise that this is done by ambulatory blood pressure monitoring (ABPM), which means wearing a machine which checks BP at least twice per hour during a normal day. BP can be falsely high in a medical clinic (some people get stressed out by the white coats!) and often the ABPM shows that your BP is normal in your everyday life. If your clinic BP is 140/90 or above and your ABPM is an average of 135/85 or higher, then you have hypertension, and need further tests and assessment. If your clinic BP is 180/120 or higher, then you need urgent assessment and possibly an immediate specialist opinion.

Regular exercise can reduce BP by 5 to 7mmHg. When you stop exercising, BP drops to a little below its normal pressure and can remain there for 24 hours, so regular and frequent exercise is ideal to keep BP down. However, during exercise, your systolic BP initially goes up as the heart pumps harder, so if you already have a high and uncontrolled BP, then pushing it even higher with vigorous exercise, such as running, can potentially be harmful. The safest thing to do in your situation would be to avoid running until you have seen your doctor. Once your doctor has assessed you and determined whether you do indeed have hypertension, then they can advise you about the safety of running. If you have significant hypertension, then they may suggest waiting until it is under control with medication before returning to running. You can drop to low or moderate intensity exercise such as regular brisk walking in the meantime.

Q I often feel faint straight after a long run and have to sit down. Is this normal?

A This frequently happens to runners, especially when they stop abruptly at the finish line after a long-distance race. When muscles are working hard during a run they need an increased blood flow to supply them with extra oxygen and to take away the waste products they create. When you stop running suddenly, that increased blood volume can pool in your legs, making blood pressure drop. Low blood pressure is called hypotension and it leaves you feeling light-headed, dizzy and at risk of fainting. If this happens to you, then lie down immediately (where it's safe to do so) and raise your legs above the level of your heart. Alternatively, you can crouch or sit down with your head between your knees. Have a drink – preferably a rehydration sports drink containing electrolytes and carbohydrates in case dehydration and low sugar levels are adding to your faintness. Allow yourself at least 10 minutes to recover and then get up slowly, moving to sitting before you stand as you may find your blood pressure falls again on being upright. To avoid this situation, make sure you don't stop running abruptly. Keep moving when you cross the finish line. Have a warm-down jog or a brisk walk for five to 10 minutes to allow your body to slowly adjust to the reduced demands on it.

Q I've been getting a few palpitations from time to time. Is it dangerous for me to run?

A The term palpitations is used to describe a sensation that your heart is beating stronger, louder or faster than normal or that it seems to be missing beats or jumping around irregularly. The first thing to determine is whether your palpitations are harmful or not. Palpitations are common, usually harmless and tend to resolve with lifestyle changes such as reducing caffeine, alcohol and stress.

Feeling excited, anxious or scared can cause your heart to thump rapidly in your chest. This can feel unpleasant, but isn't harmful. If your heart seems to be missing a beat, then this may be harmless too. When the heart's electrical activity gets briefly out of sync a beat can come a little early and then there's a pause before the next one. These are called ectopic beats and are common.

However, there are several warning signs that might indicate your palpitations are more serious. If you experience chest pain or tightness, are very short of breath or faint with your palpitations, then this is a medical emergency and you need to dial 999 for an ambulance. Palpitations that are triggered by exercise or make you feel nauseated, dizzy or out of breath need to be urgently investigated to check for an underlying cause.

If you don't have any other symptoms but your palpitations are happening on most days, last longer than a few minutes or your pulse is jumping around in an irregular rhythm (whether it's fast or slow), then you need to see a doctor for investigations. Unless your doctor is confident that these are 'benign' palpitations, they will arrange for you to have some blood tests, an ECG (heart tracing) and possibly an ECG which you wear for 24 to 72 hours. The medical causes of palpitations are numerous and include abnormal heart rhythms such as atrial fibrillation (see page 47), heart block, underlying heart disease, anaemia, an overactive thyroid and hormonal changes such as the menopause.

If there are no warning signs with your palpitations and they don't occur when you're exercising, then going for a run is unlikely to be dangerous. If you have any concerns or other symptoms, then hold off the running until you have been assessed.

Q How do I know if the pain in my chest is coming from my heart?

A It can be impossible to tell. Typical heart pain is a pain felt in the centre of the chest. It's often described as a dull pain, like a heavy pressure on the chest or a tight band around it. There might be associated symptoms such as pallor, nausea, sweating or palpitations. Pains that originate from the lungs are usually sharper, worse on breathing in or coughing, and cause more shortness of breath. However, and this is important, we don't all conform to text book descriptions. Heart pain may present in different ways, particularly in women.

Heart pain happens when the cardiac muscle isn't getting adequate blood supply, so it's more likely to happen when you are stressing the heart with exercise. Any chest pain that comes on when you are exerting yourself should be checked by a doctor. If the pain is sudden, severe, spreading to your arms, neck or jaw and not easing after 15 minutes, then it could be a heart attack and you should dial 999. There are many other causes of chest pain, such as indigestion, anxiety and muscular pain, but it's always best to have heart pain excluded, so make an appointment with your doctor if you are concerned.

Q I get really cold, white fingers when I run in the winter. My gran says it's bad circulation.

A Your gran is partly right. This sounds like Raynaud's Disease.
There is plenty of blood reaching your hands, so there is
nothing wrong with your circulation per se, but what happens
in Raynaud's is that the tiny blood vessels in your fingers constrict and
spasm in response to the cold, reducing blood flow. This can happen
to toes, ears and noses too. It can be very frustrating for runners,
especially during the winter months, because as well as turning white
and blue, fingers can go numb, making pressing sports watch buttons
or retying shoe laces really tricky. It can also be painful when the blood
returns to the fingers as they warm up again. The best bet is to try to
stop your hands getting cold in the first place with insulated gloves,
glove liners and warmers, and making sure your whole body is warm.

Q Can I exercise with varicose veins?

A Varicose veins are swollen veins near the surface of the skin.
They can be straight or wiggly, narrow or wide and are dark blue
in colour. They may not cause any symptoms at all but sometimes
they can ache, throb, itch or even bleed. Varicose veins develop when

blood backs up in a vein. This usually happen when the valves inside the vein, which are designed to prevent back-flow of blood, become weak. Valves weaken with age but being overweight or spending lots of time on your feet increases your risk too. The changing female hormones during pregnancy and the menopause cause relaxation of the vein walls which can make them swell. There's often a genetic link too so you might be able to blame your parents for your varicose veins.

Exercise helps to reduce the chance of developing varicose veins and you shouldn't stop exercising if you develop them. Regular exercise is an important part of treatment. It works the lower leg muscles which act as a pump, pushing blood back up the veins to the heart. If your legs ache or your varicose veins are more swollen, painful or tender after exercise then it's a sign you have done too much. Elevate your legs for half an hour to ease any discomfort. Off-road running can be more comfortable than high-impact road running. There's little evidence that low grade sports compression socks will stop varicose veins getting any worse but they may make you feel more comfortable. If you knock a delicate vein it may bleed. Don't be alarmed. Elevate your leg and press firmly over the bleeding point with a clean cloth. If the bleeding doesn't seem to be reducing after a few minutes then seek medical help.

Q I gave blood yesterday. Can I run today?

A It's best to wait 24 hours after donating. You can then run if you feel OK, but do bear in mind that you have donated just under a pint of blood, which is 10 per cent of your total blood volume. The body quickly tops up the plasma (fluid) in your bloodstream to maintain your blood pressure, but the red blood cells, which are required to transport oxygen around the body, can take six to 12 weeks to return to normal levels. Try a short, easy run and see how you go. If you feel weak, light-headed or out of breath, then take a few days' rest, drink plenty of fluids and eat iron-rich foods to help red blood cell formation. Remember that your performance will be affected for two to three weeks after you've given blood, so plan your donations during the recovery time after a race rather than in the weeks before. It's also useful to know that the blood service ask that you don't do strenuous exercise just before you donate. This is to ensure you are well hydrated and rested to prevent light headedness during donation and help you recover more quickly afterwards.

Real-life runners

I gave my 30th blood donation and decided that the half marathon three days later would be OK if I just went steady. The wheels came off at nine miles into the Conwy Half Marathon. My energy drained away totally. I found myself jogging slowly back, being passed by all my club mates, who looked puzzled as to why I was so much slower than usual. The last four miles seemed to take about a week to cover...

Graeme, UKA group leader, co-founder of Crewe parkrun

Did you know?

It's the haemoglobin in red blood cells that gives them their red colour. Normal levels for a male are 130-180g/L and 115-165g/L for a female.

Q I've heard running can give you low iron levels. Should all runners take iron supplements?

A Iron is essential for the high demands of running. It's not uncommon for athletes to be deficient in iron, which can have a negative effect on performance. You would assume, therefore, that all runners should take iron. There are situations where iron supplements are a good idea, but there are others where this may be harmful. If we explore the theory behind it, things become clearer.

Iron is required to make haemoglobin, the component of the red blood cell which carries oxygen around the body. Red blood cells are made in the bone marrow. Each red cell survives about 100 days, so new ones are constantly being produced. When red blood cell numbers drop below a certain level, then a person is said to be anaemic. You can become anaemic for two reasons: either you aren't making enough red blood cells or the red blood cells are being used up too quickly. Thankfully conditions of the bone marrow, where red cell production occurs, are rare. You're more likely to be anaemic due to a shortage of the ingredients for making red blood cells and the most common cause of anaemia in the UK is iron deficiency. Either your diet is low in iron or your body is not absorbing iron from foods, which can happen in conditions such as coeliac disease or inflammatory bowel disease.

If red cell production is normal, then losing blood cells more quickly than they are being made is the second explanation for anaemia. An obvious example of this is a heavy monthly period in a menstruating woman. This is a situation when taking an iron supplement is a good idea. Blood loss, however, can sometimes be subtle or silent. Blood lost in faeces or urine is a sign of potential bowel or bladder cancer and needs to be investigated. Taking an iron supplement in this situation could potentially mask the symptoms and signs of cancer, and lead to a late diagnosis.

Training intensively in any sport can put you at risk of anaemia. Whether running reduces red blood cell levels more than other sports is a little controversial. The mechanism by which it might do this is also unclear as there are conflicting studies. There is a concept called foot-strike haemolysis, where red blood cells are thought to be destroyed by being squashed when the foot hits the ground. A small study of ten male triathletes in 2003 compared the amount of red blood cell damage during one hour of cycling and running. While both activities caused some exercise-induced haemolysis, there was more haemolysis in the runners. The conclusion being that the impact from foot-strike was the major contributor to the breakdown of red blood cells during running. In contrast, a study of 18 male endurance runners after a 60-kilometre ultramarathon in 2012 didn't show significant changes in red blood cells and haemoglobin, and concluded that foot-strike haemolysis was not an important contributing factor for anaemia in athletes.

Certainly, with the high demands of regular running, your body needs a great diet to supply all the building blocks to repair and strengthen it, and if your dietary iron is insufficient then you may run yourself into trouble. Generally speaking, with a good diet there is no need for runners to take iron supplements, although if you're a menstruating woman you might choose to do so. Symptoms of anaemia include feeling tired, being out of breath on exertion and having a rapid pulse. Headaches, dizziness and looking very pale are common too. If you think you might be anaemic, or have any bowel or bladder symptoms, then don't just reach for the iron tablets. See your doctor first for investigation of the cause.

Diet tips for boosting iron

TRY THIS AT HOME

Whether you're deficient in iron or not, as a runner it's a good idea to make sure your diet is packed with iron. Here are some simple things you can do to boost your dietary iron:

- Drink a glass of orange juice with your iron-rich foods – the Vitamin C it contains helps with iron absorption.
- Snack on dried apricots, nuts and seeds.
- Remember eggs! Hard-boiled eggs can be left in their shell in the fridge for around a week – perfect for a snack or a packed lunch.
- Eat lots of leafy green vegetables. Throw a handful of spinach leaves into your salad, omelette or pasta or serve broccoli or kale with your main meal.
- Don't forget seafood and fish. We know that red meat contains lots of iron, but so do shellfish such as mussels, clams and oysters. Tinned sardines or tuna are an easy option.
- Chickpeas are your friend. Full of iron and used straight from the tin, you can throw them in salads, soups, curries and casseroles.

continued overleaf ▶

- Garnish excessively! Topping your meal with a large pile of fresh coriander, parsley or watercress adds flavour and also iron.
- Look for breakfast cereals fortified with iron.
- Cut back on tea and don't drink it with your food, because the tannin it contains inhibits iron absorption.

Q My doctor says I'm anaemic and has given me iron tablets, but said it would take a few months for my iron levels to become normal. Can I run or do I need to wait?

A You may become anaemic so gradually that you don't notice any effect on your ability to exercise. However, being anaemic can make you feel tired, out of breath and light-headed. Your heart rate is also likely to be increased as the body is pumping what red cells it has around the body as fast as possible. This obviously makes running difficult and your performance level can drop significantly. It's a classic example of a situation where it's best to listen to your body. Be guided by how you feel. If you're struggling with your breathing, or feeling exhausted or dizzy when you exercise, then you should cut back to something gentler or rest for a while. It can take several weeks for your iron levels to return to normal, so be patient and don't book any races or tough training sessions during this time. Your doctor will probably suggest that you continue the iron tablets for several weeks after your blood levels are normal, to build up your body's iron stores. Read the answer about iron supplements and remember to increase the iron in your diet too by following the diet tips.

Q My dad had a heart attack when he was 50. Does this mean I shouldn't run in case it happens to me?

A Your family's health can have a direct impact on yours, both through the genes that are passed on and through the living environments you share. The fact your dad had a heart attack doesn't mean it will definitely happen to you, but it does increase your risk. Immediate family, such as your parents and siblings, are called first degree relatives and their medical history has the biggest influence on yours. Because your dad had his heart attack when he was less than 55 years old (it would be less than 65 if it was your mum), then you are classed as having a strong family history of heart disease and we know this puts you at increased risk.

You can't change your genetics, but you can change your environment through making healthy lifestyle choices. Family history is only one risk factor for heart disease. Others include smoking, type 2 diabetes, high blood pressure, high cholesterol and being inactive or overweight. Remember that regular exercise such as running is a very powerful tool for reducing all of these risk factors.

Your family history certainly doesn't mean that you shouldn't run, but it would be sensible for you to take some steps to have your personal risk formally assessed. If you are aged between 40 and 74 then you can have this done during an NHS health check at your local GP practice. Your blood pressure, weight, blood cholesterol and blood sugar will be checked to help identify risk factors that need treatment, and you will be given lots of advice. If you have never run before, due to your strong family history, I suggest a check before you begin. However, if you are already running regularly then don't stop, but make a routine appointment.

Q Why do some people die suddenly in marathons? What are the risks?

A death during a marathon is always tragic, but be reassured that it is rare. The *New England Journal of Medicine* published a study in 2012 assessing cardiac arrests during marathons and half marathons in the USA between 2000 and 2010. In the races studied there were 10.9 million runners and 59 cardiac arrests, 42 of which were fatal. This means that approximately one person in 260,000 died from a cardiac arrest in the population studied. According to a table of everyday risks in the *British Journal of Medicine*, we have a one in 250,000 risk of being hit in our own home by a crashing aeroplane. There were more cardiac arrests in the marathons than the half marathons and more in men than women. Most of the cardiac arrests were due to cardiovascular disease (more common in the older runners) and to hypertrophic cardiomyopathy (HOCM). This is an inherited condition where the heart wall becomes thickened. There are often symptoms of breathlessness, palpitations and chest pain, but it's a common cause of sudden cardiac death in those under 35 years old. If a diagnosis of HOCM is made, then genetic testing and screening may be offered to close relatives. Some sporting organisations screen their young athletes for HOCM. Remember that not all cardiac conditions that cause sudden death can be detected.

A narrative review of the literature, including the study above, was published in a journal called *BMJ Open* in 2019. It looked at deaths during or within 24 hours of completing a marathon (no other race distances were included). This found the risk of death to be approximately one per 102,000 in men and one per 244,000 in women. The conclusion was that the risk of death from participating in a marathon is small, higher for men and greatest in the final few miles of the race.

First aid

Consider going on a first aid course to learn basic life support. A few hours of your time could save a life in the future. Find a course near you and book a place. St John's Ambulance runs first aid courses up and down the country.

TRY THIS AT HOME

Q What should I do if the runner in front of me during a race collapses?

 Stay calm and follow these basic life support steps:

1 **Check it's safe.** Look after yourself first. Don't trip yourself or others up in a bid to reach the casualty.
2 **Call for help.** Shout to other runners or a nearby marshal to help you.
3 **Talk to the runner.** Perhaps they've just gone down with a severe leg cramp rather than a cardiac arrest. If they can talk and tell you what's going on, then you can assist them to get the help they need. If they're talking but delirious and not making sense, then lie them on their side in the recovery position. Keep talking to them while you summon medical help. Ask them if they have any medical conditions and check the back of their running bib or any medical alert jewellery (bracelets, shoe tags or necklaces) for this information too.
4 **Check for breathing.** If they aren't responding when you talk loudly and directly to their face while gently shaking them, then they are unconscious and this is an emergency. You need to see if they are breathing normally, so roll them onto their back and open their airway by gently tipping their head back with one hand and lifting their chin with the other. Now LOOK, LISTEN and FEEL for signs of breathing for up to 10 seconds. If they are

breathing normally, then put them in the recovery position and keep checking them while you call and wait for the paramedics.

5 **If they aren't breathing normally.** If they are unconscious and not breathing normally, then there are three things that need to happen:

- You need to dial 999 and state that the casualty is not breathing.
- You need to locate an AED (Automated External Defibrillator). The emergency services call handler will tell you where one is located if you don't know. Race marshals may be able to radio to base to summon one.
- You need to start chest compressions.

If you are on your own, then carry out these steps in this order. Defibrillation is the priority. If you have people around you that can help, then all three can happen simultaneously. You can tell someone to call an ambulance and another to get an AED while you commence chest compressions. Put your phone on speaker mode and the emergency call handler will talk you through it.

There may be someone at hand who is experienced in resuscitation, in which case let them take the lead. Chest compressions (at a rate of 100 to 120 per minute) are more important than rescue breaths, but if you feel able and comfortable to give rescue breaths then briefly stop chest compressions every 30 compressions to give two breaths.

Remember CPR (cardiopulmonary resuscitation) is tiring and you may already be exhausted from your running, so swap and take turns with others to maintain the quality of the chest compressions.

Just do your best – it's better than no CPR at all. If the AED arrives before the paramedics, then use it by following the instructions on the package and the verbal instructions when you turn it on. AEDs will only shock if necessary, so don't be afraid to use one. They save lives.

Continue until the ambulance arrives. If the casualty starts breathing again in the meantime, then put them in the recovery position.

A shock from a defibrillator within one minute of collapse gives a 90 per cent chance of survival. For every minute after that, the chance reduces by 7 to 10 per cent. Speed is of the essence.

Q I run a lot of marathons and ultras. Will this damage my heart in the long term?

A Running is definitely good for your heart, but there is probably a point at which too much running can cause harm. What that exact tipping point is, however, is unknown and most certainly different for each individual. The effect endurance exercise will have on our body depends on many variables, including our gender, race, age, training methods and our body's DNA.

We know that athletes' hearts can look different to non-athletes'. Vigorous and repetitive training induces changes called cardiac remodelling. The chambers of the heart can become enlarged due to the sustained high volumes of blood passing through them. There are similar changes evident in life-threatening cardiac disorders, but there's no evidence that the changes are harmful in athletes. Interestingly, there may be less cardiac remodelling in women, but there's not enough evidence to confirm that yet. As more and more women are participating in endurance sports there is certainly more research to come.

One of the other changes that is seen in the hearts of endurance athletes is myocardial fibrosis. This is patchy scarring in the heart muscle, but its significance is unclear. A study of 12 life-long, veteran, male endurance athletes was carried out in 2011. When their hearts were compared to non-athletes of the same age and to younger endurance athletes too, 50 per cent of the veteran athletes were found to have some degree of myocardial fibrosis. There was none in the non-athletes or younger men. This suggests a link between life-long endurance exercise and myocardial fibrosis, but the endurance athletes were all fit and well with no cardiac symptoms, so perhaps the changes are harmless. It has been suggested that myocardial fibrosis is a cause of atrial fibrillation (AF). This is the most common cause of a persistently irregular pulse and it requires medical treatment, because it is associated with an increased risk of stroke. In AF, the electrical activity which triggers the cardiac muscle of the atria to contract becomes uncoordinated. Rather than having one distinct squeeze, the atria quivers and fibrillates, which makes it inefficient at pumping blood to the ventricle.

A review published in the *British Journal of Sports Medicine* examined nearly 50 years of medical literature and confirmed that endurance athletes, particularly older ones, have an increased risk of AF. There were many suggested causes for this. Studies to date have focused on long-term endurance athletes, but there may be a completely different story for the average recreational athlete who does intermittent endurance events.

TOP TIPS FOR A HEALTHY RUNNER'S HEART

- Don't smoke.
- Exercise regularly. Aim for at least 150 minutes of moderate intensity activity per week. Running counts as vigorous activity, so only 75 minutes per week is required.
- Maintain a normal weight.
- Eat a healthy, varied diet full of fresh vegetables and oily fish, and avoid excess salt.
- Get your blood pressure checked at least every five years (unless you have hypertension or other medical conditions that require more frequent checks).
- Prioritise recovery on your training plan.
- Reduce your stress levels.
- Reduce sedentary time – move frequently and don't rely on running as your only exercise.
- Don't race with a viral illness.
- Listen to your body.

FURTHER HELP AND ADVICE

NICE guidelines: www.nice.org.uk
British Heart Foundation: www.bhf.org.uk
Scleroderma and Raynaud's UK: www.sruk.co.uk
Giving blood: www.blood.co.uk
NHS What's your heart age?: www.nhs.uk
First aid advice and courses – St John's Ambulance: www.sja.org.uk
Resuscitation Council UK: www.resus.org.uk
BDA: The Association of UK Dieticians: www.bda.uk.com
Cardiac Risk in the Young: www.c-r-y.org.uk

CHAPTER 3

THE RESPIRATORY SYSTEM

All runners know how it feels to be out of breath. Whether you're a beginner taking your first running steps or an experienced runner tackling a tough hill repeats session, you know how difficult it is to keep going when your lungs feel as if they're about to explode. Running is a great way to strengthen our lungs and increase our lung capacity, so in this chapter we'll explore some of the lung issues that runners come up against. We'll also take a look at problems affecting the nose and sinuses as these are part of the respiratory system too.

The main function of the respiratory system is to bring oxygen into the body and take carbon dioxide and other waste gases out. There are approximately 1500 miles of airways in our lungs (this is the equivalent of flying from London to Moscow). The journey begins in the nose or mouth where air enters and flows into the trachea, commonly known as the windpipe. This then splits into the right and left main bronchi, which further divide and branch into smaller bronchi, then even smaller bronchioles, where gas transfer takes place in 300 to 500 million microscopic alveoli. It's here in the alveoli where oxygen diffuses into the blood to re-oxygenate it and waste gases, including carbon dioxide, diffuse out. When you breathe out the waste gases are emptied from the body and water vapour is lost too, which is why you can see your breath when you exhale on a cold morning run.

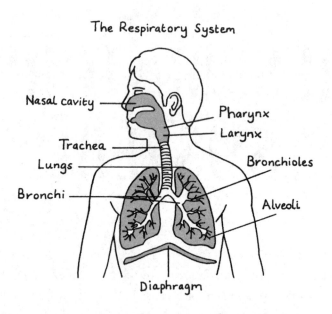

The Respiratory System

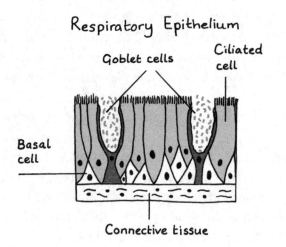

Respiratory Epithelium

Our airways are lined with a special tissue called the respiratory epithelium. This tissue protects us from dirt particles and germs and keeps our airways moist and healthy. The four main types of cell making up this lining tissue are:

- **Ciliated cells** These line the trachea and bronchi. Each cell has around 200 cilia (microscopic legs) on its surface, which it waves repeatedly to transport mucous up towards the mouth.
- **Goblet cells** Shaped like a wine goblet, these cells produce mucous to trap dirt and germs.
- **Basal cells** These small cells are the reserve bench, and can step up and change into any type of respiratory cell, depending on what is needed to keep the epithelium healthy.
- **Alveolar cells** These are found in the lining of the alveoli and are specially designed for gas transfer.

Surrounding the respiratory epithelium you'll find loose connective tissue containing blood vessels, elastic fibres and smooth muscle. This smooth muscle is under the control of the parasympathetic nervous system, which means we can't control its contraction or relaxation. Although not strictly part of the respiratory system, we need to acknowledge the ribs, which protect the lungs, and the chest muscles and diaphragm, which allow the lungs to expand and contract.

Did you know?

The surface area of your lungs is approximately the size of a tennis court.

The respiratory system is incredible. It ensures that we breathe clean air, deliver it to the bloodstream and get rid of waste products, all in the blink of an eye. As runners, we really put the system to the test and showcase its power, so it's easy to see how a small issue in one part of the system can cause problems and upset the process.

Q Should I breathe through my nose or mouth when I run?

A When you first start running you're very aware of your breath, mostly because you can't seem to catch it! As your fitness increases you can take slow runs while holding a good conversation and not actually think about your breathing at all. You probably don't even know whether you nose- or mouth-breathe! Next time you're out for a run, observe your breathing. Most of us mouth-breathe. There is much debate about the 'right' way to breathe when you run, with some running coaches saying you should breathe through your nose, others saying your mouth, and others saying a combination of in through your nose and out through your mouth is best.

A small but interesting study tested 10 runners who had been nasal breathing while exercising for six months. They put them through a series of tests, first while breathing through their nose and then while mouth-only breathing. Runners generally complain that they can't get enough air in if they try to breathe through their nose, but it is something that takes practice to master. The nose allows air to be warmed before it reaches the lungs and the mucous and hairs in the nasal passages filter out pathogens and particles, so potentially it's beneficial to breathe in through your nose. The subjects in this study took in the same amount of oxygen during both nasal and mouth breathing, but when they were nose breathing, their breathing rate was slower and their breath more economical. It is certainly easier to relax while nose breathing as it forces you to breathe more slowly. Other studies, however, have pointed out that although breathing rate is slower while nasal breathing, the heart rate can be higher, putting stress on the body in a different way. Without clear evidence either way it seems that personal preference is best, but do familiarise yourself with diaphragmatic breathing (see page 59).

Q Why does my nose run when I do?

A This is a very common problem. A runny nose or rhinitis, to use its medical name, can be triggered by a number of things. Obviously, your nose runs if a virus, such as the common cold, irritates it, but the same thing can happen when it's exposed to dust, pollen, pollution, chemicals or cold air. Sometimes a runny nose is triggered purely by exercise itself and this is called exercise-induced rhinitis. Nasal mucous does have its purpose, though. It's not simply produced to annoy us! It protects us by stopping dirt, dust and germs entering our system as we breathe in rapidly during running. The slightly frustrating thing is that when you run, your body is trying to get as much oxygen as possible into your lungs, so your nostrils flare and nasal passages open up, allowing more air (and more irritant) in with every inhalation.

Work out what your trigger is and then try to avoid or minimise your exposure to it. This might involve avoiding running beside queueing traffic, or covering your nose with a light scarf to warm the cold air before you breathe it in or to stop pollen reaching your nose.

Make a trip to your local pharmacist – there is a range of products for rhinitis that can be bought over the counter. These include nasal sprays containing decongestants, antihistamines or corticosteroids. Oral (tablet or liquid) antihistamines are also useful. Your pharmacist will advise you which would be best for you. You could also try nasal irrigation, which means washing out your

Did you know?

Your respiratory tract produces more than a litre of mucous per day!

nasal passages with salty water. Again, the pharmacist can advise you on how to do this. Rhinitis that doesn't improve with treatment or involves smelly or blood-stained nasal discharge (particularly from one side) should always be checked by a doctor. Some winter gloves have an absorbent pad for wiping away the snot or you can shove a tissue in your pocket, use your sleeve or master the 'snot rocket', but please check there isn't anyone behind you!

Q Hay fever destroys my summer running. Do you have any tips on managing it?

A The hay fever season can extend from March to October for some people, depending on which pollens trigger their symptoms. Itchy, watery eyes, a runny nose and sneezing are the usual symptoms, but hay fever can also cause coughing and wheezing, particularly in people who have asthma. In the UK, you can visit the Met Office daily pollen forecast online and avoid running on days when the count is at its highest or opt to run indoors on a treadmill instead (remember to keep the windows closed). The count is likely to be lowest on cooler days, during and after rain, and when there isn't too much wind to blow the pollen around, so get your trainers on and head out when these days appear.

When you do run, try to reduce the amount of pollen reaching your face. A hat with a brim, wraparound sunglasses and a light scarf to cover your mouth will all help. Try dabbing some petroleum jelly just at the entrance to your nostrils to trap pollen. When you've finished running, shower straight away, and wash your hair and your running kit to remove the pollen. Dry your running kit indoors to avoid it getting coated with pollen. As with a runny nose (rhinitis), there are plenty of medications you can buy from the pharmacy to ease and prevent hay fever symptoms. You can direct treatment at the worst affected area, for example eye drops for itchy eyes and a nasal spray for sneezing, or you can take oral antihistamines to work throughout the body. Sometimes you need a combination of both, but your pharmacist can advise you. If hay fever is upsetting your asthma control, then make an appointment with your asthma nurse or GP for an assessment.

 ## Will running will help my asthma?

The belief that people with asthma shouldn't exercise has long been discarded – we now have plenty of evidence that exercise helps asthma. A review in 2013 looked at 21 studies involving asthma and exercise (including running), and found no adverse effects on the participants' asthma from exercising. In fact, there was an improvement in cardiopulmonary (heart and lung) fitness and an improved health-related quality of life too. Another review of the literature, published in the *Journal of Asthma* also in 2013, found that regular exercise improved the management of asthma symptoms, lung function and mental health, and that inactive people with asthma had more asthma-related difficulties. So regular exercise is an important part of a healthy lifestyle for people with asthma. However, if at any point you have difficult-to-control or severe asthma, then it's essential that you speak to your health care team before you exercise.

Real-life runners

Running quickly for long periods of time hasn't been easy for me with asthma. However, when I slow my pace and keep it relaxed and steady, I find I can run amazing distances that I never thought possible! The cold weather can cause me to cough, but I usually still run, and after I have warmed up it tends to calm down. I also find a neck scarf and thermal layers are really helpful in preventing symptoms on cold days.

Abi Chapman, runner and mum

Q What's the best way to stop running triggering my asthma symptoms?

A Make sure you attend regularly for asthma checks with your nurse or doctor, even if you feel well. These are an opportunity to have your lung function checked, talk through any symptoms you are having and make sure you remain on the most appropriate treatment. Your nurse or doctor will also devise an asthma action plan so you feel confident about how to manage your asthma between checks and know exactly when you should seek help or further treatment.

Exercise is a common trigger for asthma, especially during hay fever season or in the winter months, when cold dry air can bring on symptoms. Adequate treatment should mean that you are able to exercise freely, although you may have to step up your treatment plan to keep good control during the times of year that you find hardest. Your 'preventer' inhalers (usually brown) are the mainstay of your treatment. They reduce inflammation in the lungs and stop symptoms occurring in the first place, so it's vital to take these regularly. You should always carry your 'reliever' inhaler (usually blue) with you when you run, but it isn't necessary to take it before you set off. Include a good warm-up and cool-down as part of your run to gradually get your lungs used to the change of exertion. See the tips on avoiding exposure to triggers in the question on hay fever above, but the trick of warming the air you breathe by covering your mouth and nose with a light scarf is really helpful for winter running with asthma. If you feel your asthma is not fully under control, for example if you have a viral infection, then don't run and follow the steps in your personalised asthma action plan.

Did you know?

The right lung is bigger than the left lung, because the left lung has a 'cardiac notch' carved out of it to make space for the heart.

Q I'm OK normally, but I seem to get wheezy and cough when I get home afterwards. Do I have asthma?

A You may have heard the term 'exercise-induced asthma' (EIA), it refers to asthmatic symptoms, such as coughing, wheezing or chest tightness, which occur during or, more often, after exercise. It is sometimes referred to as 'exercise-induced bronchospasm' (EIB), describing the way the bronchi (small airways in the lungs) spasm and narrow in response to exercise. These two terms, EIA and EIB, are often used interchangeably, but there is debate as to whether they are the same thing, what causes each one and ultimately what is the best way to treat them.

A runner with EIA gets symptoms because they have underlying asthma and exercise is the trigger. A runner with EIB gets symptoms despite not necessarily having asthma. The American College of Allergy, Asthma and Immunology states that as many as 90 per cent of people with asthma also have EIB, but not everyone with EIB has asthma. EIB is more common in cold weather sports, such as skiing and ice skating, and in endurance running. The exact cause of EIB is unknown, but it is thought that heavy breathing during exercise causes the airways to dry out. This dehydration then triggers a range of chemical substances to be released in the lungs, which leads to inflammation and airway narrowing. Reliever (usually blue) inhalers such as salbutamol stop airway spasm by relaxing the smooth muscle in the lining of the airways, allowing them to open up. This is an ideal first treatment for EIB and salbutamol can be used 15 minutes before a run to help prevent it. However, if the underlying cause is more complicated and involves any inflammation, which may be the case in EIB and is certainly a component of EIA, then treatment with preventer meds such as inhaled corticosteroids need to be considered.

It's tricky for the GP that sees you with your exercise-induced cough or wheeze! Advanced lung testing to determine the exact cause of your symptoms isn't readily available for recreational athletes, and usually it's a case of exploring your history and symptoms to determine whether you may have an underlying asthma, and monitoring your response to treatment. This is clearly not ideal, so don't be afraid to make a further appointment with your GP if your symptoms aren't improving, but read on as there may be another cause too.

Q Sometimes when I run I can feel my throat closing up and I can't get enough air in. My breathing is very noisy and wheezy. It happens mostly when I race and I've had to pull out as I just can't breathe.

A It's often assumed that all wheezing and breathing symptoms when you exercise come from the lungs, but this isn't always the case. There is a condition called Exercise Induced Laryngeal Obstruction (EILO) that is increasingly being diagnosed, but is still often overlooked. The larynx is your voice box and during intense exercise it can sometimes become narrowed. We don't really understand why this happens, but the delicate folds of tissue in the larynx close in, partially blocking the airway and leading to a noisy, wheezy inward breath as air tries to squeeze past. It is more common in young, adolescent athletes. Currently, the only definite way to diagnose it is to look at the larynx with a fibre optic laryngoscope (a small camera on a tube that goes up the nose and down the throat) while the patient is exercising at full speed on a treadmill or rowing machine. You may also hear the term Vocal Cord Dysfunction (VCD) to describe this phenomenon, but the narrowing really occurs above the vocal cords. EILO doesn't respond to the (blue) reliever inhalers such as salbutamol used in EIB. Instead, treatment centres on behavioural management with a speech and language specialist. Techniques involve relaxing the neck and throat muscles, learning breathing techniques for when the symptoms start, and identifying and managing triggers such as stress, which might account for increased symptoms during races. If you think you may have EILO then discuss your suspicions with your GP who will be able to refer you to a specialist for investigation.

Real-life runners

During races and training I was finding it really hard to breathe, as if I couldn't get any air in at all. I discovered that this happened when I was stressed. Since I learnt how to calm my breathing down it has been fine.

Steven, junior athlete and cross-country runner

Diaphragmatic breathing

TRY THIS AT HOME

The diaphragm is a sheet of muscle beneath our lungs, dividing our chest cavity from our abdominal cavity. Its contraction and relaxation creates and releases a vacuum, which pulls air in and out of the lungs. Many of us, however, tend to use our upper chest muscles to drive our breathing. By focusing on and maximising our diaphragmatic breathing we can ensure that we're getting the most out of each breath, which can potentially help our performance. If you observe a young baby, you'll see their belly blowing in and out as they breathe. This is what we need to try to relearn.

- Lie on your back and place the flat palm of your hand on your abdomen, just below your rib cage.
- Take a breath in. As you do so, try to keep your shoulders and chest still, and use that breath to blow out your belly. You should see your hand moving upwards.
- As you exhale, watch your hand sinking back down again.
- Repeat this for 20 breaths or until you want to stop.

When you've mastered this technique lying down, you can try it sitting, standing and eventually running. When you do it, always make sure you have good posture and are standing tall with your shoulders back. Complete a session of diaphragmatic breathing every day and gradually it will become natural. Spending some time quietly focusing on breathing in this way is also a great relaxation technique.

Q Is it OK to run with a cold? I get one every winter and don't want to miss training.

A It can be really hard to maintain training right throughout the main cold and cough season. When a respiratory infection strikes, it's usually a virus and your airways respond by producing more mucous – which makes you feel very stuffed up, affects your breathing and can make you cough. The mucous may all come from your upper airways, drip down the back of your throat and produce a wet sounding cough, but sometimes the cough is dry and makes your throat feel sore. People often assume that the greener the mucous, the nastier the infection, but we now know this isn't true and both bacterial and viral infections of differing severity (and even allergies too) can result in clear, yellow, green or brown mucous.

The key really is how does your breathing feel and how are you in yourself? If you just have a bit of a runny nose, sneezing and a dry, tickly cough, then you're unlikely to do any harm by having a gentle run. In fact, exercise may help to relieve your nasal congestion and make you feel a little better in the short term. Don't push it, though. Take it easy and see how you feel. If, however, you are more out of breath than normal (test this out by walking up a set of stairs), have any chest pains, or are wheezing or coughing repeatedly, then you really shouldn't run. Similarly, if you have a high temperature, feel nauseated, achy or just fatigued, then stressing your body by running is not advised. It's far better to allow a few extra days to get properly well and then return to training (see page 201 for more advice on running and illness).

Did you know?

Vital capacity is the amount of air you can breathe out after you've taken a deep breath in. It's basically a measure of your lung volume. It varies with gender, age, race and height, but it's between three and five litres.

Q I keep hearing about VO2 max. What is it and is it helpful for runners?

A Exercise requires oxygen. When you're running, your muscles demand it at a very high rate. The maximum amount of oxygen that your body can transport and use is called your VO2 max. It's a marker of your cardiovascular fitness and capacity for performance. It's measured in millilitres per kilogram of bodyweight per minute and VO2 max varies with gender, age and fitness. An inactive woman might have a VO2 max around 30ml/kg/min and an inactive man around 40ml/kg/min. Elite athletes tend to have VO2 max in the region of 60 to 85ml/kg/min with men, on average, reaching higher levels than women.

Many sports watches calculate your VO2 max for you, based on your gender, age and heart rate measurements from previous runs. These calculations aren't terribly accurate, but they give you some idea. To truly find out your own VO2 max you need to be tested on a treadmill or static bike in a laboratory while wearing a mask to measure the gas concentrations in the air you breathe in and out. You will have to exercise until you reach the point of exhaustion so be prepared to work hard! Plenty of laboratories around the country offer this service to recreational runners.

You can increase your VO2 max through training, but your upper limit is largely determined by your genetics. As your VO2 max increases you will feel fitter, be able to run faster and longer, and you will find running easier. Running sessions that increase your VO2 max include running intervals of two to three minutes at a very fast pace and then allowing three to five minutes to recover before repeating. Hill repeats are good, but rather than a short, sharp hill, find one that takes you about two to three minutes to run up. Run down slowly to recover. Cycling and rowing are great for increasing VO2 max if you work hard or you can try some HIIT (High Intensity Interval Training) too.

Whether you are interested in your VO2 max is a very personal thing. Some runners love numbers and stats, and like to track their progress, while others are just happy knowing that they feel fitter as a result of putting in some hard work.

Breathing and running

TRY THIS AT HOME

Whatever stage of running you're at, your breathing is a useful, tech-free way to monitor your effort level. It can tell you how much you're exerting yourself and you can use it to vary your intensity of effort as part of your training programme, without repeatedly looking at your watch. There are variations in definitions of the following running terms, but these are what I use as a guide. Your breathing will be faster with each one.

- **The speed of chat** You can breathe comfortably and hold a conversation. Great for sociable runs and for very long, slow runs when you're building up the miles for an endurance event.
- **Tempo pace** A tempo run is faster than your chatty run and although your breathing may take a while to calm down, it settles into a nice regular rhythm at a pace that you can sustain for about an hour. You won't want to chat away, but you could manage a few sentences. A good pace for a 40 to 60-minute training run.
- **Threshold pace** This is a 'tipping point' pace. Creep above it and your lactate levels (waste products of exercise) rise sharply and you won't be able to run for long. Stay just on it and your body is stretched, but you're able to tolerate the lactate levels and therefore the pace. You're on the edge of discomfort, but you can still keep going. Your breathing is fast, but you're able to speak a few words in a row. It's faster than a normal run, but slower than your 5km pace. With practice, you can maintain threshold pace for up to 30 minutes, so it's great to throw some threshold runs and intervals into your training if you're looking to get fitter and faster.

continued overleaf ▶

Sprint pace A super-fast pace for short distances. There's no talking on this one and you'll almost certainly be mouth-breathing at a very fast rate. You can't sustain it for more than a couple of minutes, so short sprints mixed with recovery periods during which you normalise your breathing work well.

Q I often get sinusitis. I usually just keep running through it and sometimes this seems to help.

A Sinuses are hollow air spaces in your facial bones, the main ones being the frontal sinuses (in your forehead) and the maxillary sinuses (in your cheeks). They are lined with respiratory epithelium (see page 50) that produces mucous which drains away through small passages into the nose and throat. When sinuses become inflamed it's called sinusitis – 'itis' is the Greek word for inflammation. This can happen because of infection, which is usually viral, more rarely bacterial or even fungal. It can also be triggered by allergies. Sometimes cold air can aggravate sinuses too. Commonly, sinusitis is a one-off event, usually following a cold. This is called acute sinusitis, but if it lasts more than 12 weeks it's called chronic sinusitis and other causes such as nasal polyps (non-cancerous growths) need to be considered. When the sinuses become inflamed and swollen, the holes draining the mucous away get blocked and mucous builds up in the sinuses, causing facial pressure, tenderness and congestion. Sinusitis can also cause a headache, toothache or earache and a sore throat. It may make you feel tired, dizzy and sometimes, with acute sinusitis, feverish.

When you run, adrenalin causes some of the small blood vessels in your body, such as those in your sinuses, to contract. With less blood flow to the area, the tissues become less plump and swollen and this may temporarily reduce your nasal congestion. Of course, the exercise itself can give you a feeling of wellbeing too. However, if you don't feel well in yourself, can't breathe properly or have a fever, then you shouldn't run. Thankfully, viral sinusitis usually clears on its own within three weeks. You can use pain killers, decongestants and steaming to ease your symptoms. To steam, simply fill a sink with very hot water. Make a tent by placing a towel over your head. Inhale the hot, trapped, moist air. You can add some menthol crystals or a few drops of olbas oil to make it more effective. Have a chat with your pharmacist about whether nasal steroids or antihistamines might benefit you. Chronic or recurrent sinusitis and symptoms that are just on one side of the face should be assessed by a GP, because a referral for further investigation might be needed.

Did you know?

The urge to breathe is mainly driven by rising carbon dioxide levels in the blood rather than by low oxygen levels. Sensors in the brain, and in the aorta and carotid arteries (major blood vessels), monitor levels and adjust breathing rate accordingly.

TOP TIPS FOR HEALTHY RUNNER'S LUNGS

- Don't smoke and avoid passive smoking too.
- Maintain a normal weight.
- Exercise regularly at a variety of paces.
- Eat a healthy, varied diet.
- Practise diaphragmatic breathing (see page 59).
- Avoid rush hour running to minimise exposure to air pollutants if you experience symptoms or have lung problems.
- Maintain a good running posture (see page 167) to allow your lungs to expand freely.
- Consider Pilates to help control breathing, strengthen muscles and improve posture.

FURTHER HELP AND ADVICE

Pollen counts and the Air Quality Index – Met Office: www.metoffice.gov.uk

British Lung Foundation: www.blf.org.uk

Asthma UK: www.asthma.org.uk

Allergy UK: www.allergyuk.org

British Thoracic Society guidelines: www.brit-thoracic.org.uk/quality-improvement/guidelines/

NICE guidelines: www.nice.org.uk

CHAPTER 4

THE GASTROINTESTINAL SYSTEM

O f all the body's systems, it's the gastrointestinal system that seems to cause the most frequent (and embarrassing) problems for runners. From vomiting to diarrhoea, stitches to piles, there are lots of issues that can crop up and stop you in your running tracks. But regular running has many important benefits for the gastrointestinal system, for example, helping prevent constipation and lowering your risk of bowel cancer by up to 50 per cent, so it's important to know how to overcome problems and keep going. This chapter features lots of tips and advice to make sure you're not always running towards the toilet!

The gastrointestinal system allows us to extract energy from food and get rid of waste products through digestion and excretion. Digestion begins in the mouth where food is chewed, mashed up and mixed with digestive enzymes in saliva. It's parcelled up into small packages called food boluses, which are propelled down the oesophagus (gullet) by a process called peristalsis, a series of involuntary muscular contractions. The sphincter (muscular ring) at the top of the stomach relaxes, allowing food into the stomach, where further enzymes continue to break it down and stomach acids destroy any harmful bacteria. There is a further sphincter at the bottom of the stomach which relaxes intermittently to allow small amounts of the stomach's contents to pass into the small intestine (small bowel).

The Gastrointestinal System

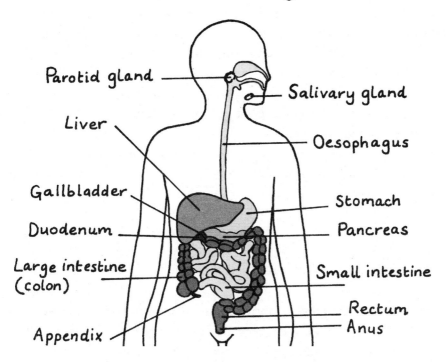

Lining of the Small Intestine

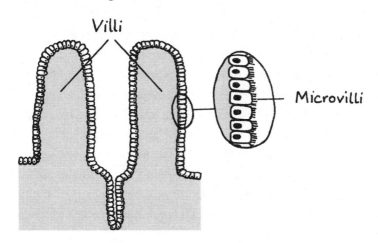

Most of the digestion and absorption of nutrients occurs in the small intestine. Food meets enzymes from the pancreas and fats are digested by bile squirted in from the gall bladder. The lining of the small intestine is specially designed to absorb nutrients into the bloodstream. It is lined with small finger like projections called villi which each have microvilli covering them. This creates a huge surface area over which nutrients can be absorbed. What's left of the food then travels on to the large intestine (large bowel), where our healthy gut bacteria break it down further and water is reabsorbed to make a formed stool. The stool is held in the rectum until the time is right for it to be expelled through the anus.

Having knowledge of our basic gut anatomy and physiology helps us to understand why things can sometimes go wrong and what we can do about them. Let's move on to answer the questions most frequently asked by runners. We'll start at the top and work our way down from mouth to anus.

Q Why do I always need to spit when I run?

Saliva is designed to lubricate our mouth and throat, and helps to keep germs out. The amount and consistency of our saliva, which is controlled by our nervous system, changes frequently. Exercise increases the flow of saliva, but also the thickness of it. Thick, sticky saliva is harder to swallow and many runners find they need to spit it out. The increase in thickness is thought to be due to a higher concentration of protein in the saliva, with moderate and vigorous exercise triggering protein production and release in the salivary glands. Cold air seems to stimulate mucous secretion too. It's also likely that water evaporates from saliva when we mouth-breathe during running and that our body produces less watery saliva if we are a bit dehydrated. All of these factors mean that we can end up with a mouthful of sticky spit and a bit of a dry mouth. There's no easy answer, but if you're particularly troubled by it then sipping small amounts of water frequently can help. Whether you think spitting is socially acceptable or not is a personal preference and you'll spark fierce debate amongst the running community if you ask that question!

Q I often get heartburn and an acid taste in my mouth when I run. Why is this and what can I do about it?

A If food and acid from your stomach travels back up your oesophagus they can give you an unpleasant tang or discomfort, usually a burning sensation, behind your breast bone. Getting a bit of acid reflux from time to time is normal, especially if you've eaten a large meal. The oesophageal sphincter sits between your oesophagus and your stomach. Its role is to prevent stomach contents from travelling back upwards, but occasionally they leak through and the acid irritates the delicate lining of the oesophagus. It's easy to see why the repetitive jiggling up and down of running might cause reflux. Eating too much, eating too close to running and not leaving enough time for digestion are obvious causes of reflux, but it's also worth seeing if there are any specific triggering foods – caffeine, fruit juices, tomatoes and spicy foods are common causes. If you're still struggling, then speak to your pharmacist about trying an antacid medication. This will neutralise the acid in your stomach and relieve the symptoms, but won't stop you getting heartburn again.

When heartburn and acid reflux are severe, happening frequently and at times when you aren't running, then you may have GORD (Gastro Oesophageal Reflux Disease). We know that being overweight, smoking and drinking alcohol can trigger GORD, so lifestyle changes to address these can help reduce symptoms, as can lowering stress levels. It's worth knowing that anti-inflammatories like ibuprofen or aspirin, commonly used by runners, can cause GORD, so you should stop these and speak to your GP. If lifestyle changes aren't controlling your symptoms, then your doctor might suggest trying medications to give you relief. These can be short or long term and are usually very effective. They might also arrange some investigations to check for underlying causes of GORD, such as a hiatus hernia, which is when part of your stomach moves up into your chest. Long term, untreated GORD can cause problems such as ulcers and in rare cases, over many years, cancer, so take action.

Q Why do I vomit when I run? It's usually after I've really pushed myself in a 10km race or during the second half of a marathon.

A 'Training till you puke' is often seen as a badge of honour, a celebration that you've pushed yourself to your limits. In all honesty, it isn't to be recommended. In short, high intensity workouts, vomiting is usually due to blood being diverted away from your gastrointestinal system and towards your skeletal muscles. Reduced blood flow to the gut slows digestion and your stomach contents then seek an alternative route out during strenuous exercise. What you've eaten and drunk before running can determine whether you vomit. Allow a couple of hours for digestion and avoid trigger foods such as citrus fruits and juices, spicy or fatty foods. If you suffer from heartburn or acid reflux, then you may be more likely to vomit during running.

Over longer distances there are more possible causes of vomiting that need to be considered. Eating on the run can make you sick, especially if you haven't practised it in training. High sugar loads from sports supplements can upset some runner's stomachs, especially if the supplements are concentrated and taken with insufficient water. Dehydration is a common cause of vomiting, but it's important to know that over-hydration can cause it too. There's a condition called hyponatraemia when the body's salt levels become dangerously low (see page 91). Don't forget that heat stroke can cause vomiting too. The dangers of heat exhaustion and heat stroke not only come from dehydration as a result of the sweat lost while running, but also from a rising core temperature (see page 217). Warming up and cooling down to avoid abrupt changes in exertion can help to prevent vomiting during and after running, so don't skimp on these if you're someone who tends to get sick!

Q After my long run I completely lose my appetite. I know I should eat, but I really don't feel like it.

A Many runners feel like this. It's thought that exercise influences the release of appetite hormones such as ghrelin, which increases appetite, and leptin, which suppresses it. This effect may vary between individuals, between men and women, and possibly between people with differing amounts of body fat. For some, a long run can reduce ghrelin and increase leptin, so you don't feel hungry at all. The 'runger' (running hunger) may not strike for several hours or even days later.

It's a good idea to ingest something after a long or hard run, but there is some doubt as to whether that magic 30-minute window to replace your glycogen stores that people talk about really exists. The ideal timing of post-exercise nutrition is debatable. Try liquids rather than solid foods if you have no appetite or feel slightly nauseated – for example, fruit smoothies, ice cold chocolate milk or a sports drink. A couple of hours later you should be ready for a more substantial feed and if you're still struggling at that point then soup is a good option. If you are listening to your body and getting the general balance between your fuelling and your running right, then you don't need to worry (see page 229).

Q What is a stitch and how can I stop it happening?

A There's a simple answer to this – we don't know! A stitch can be a dull ache, but more often it's a stabbing pain, usually in the side. It's hard to advise how to prevent it, but there are theories about what triggers it and things you can try to stop one spoiling your run. Stitches are more common in runners than they are in cyclists, which adds weight to the theory that they could be caused by the internal organs tugging on ligaments and tissues as they get jolted up and down, or by friction irritating the lining of the abdominal cavity. They're more common in beginners, runners training harder than usual and those who have eaten prior to running, so these situations suggest that a lack of blood supply to the gut or to the diaphragm muscle, resulting in cramping, may be the answer. There's also a theory that the pain isn't from the abdomen itself and originates from the spine and radiates around to the side and front. It may well be a combination of things and different for each individual. What is certain, however, is that stitches hurt and make you want to stop running!

You can try to prevent a stitch by allowing enough time for your food to be digested before you run. You'll probably need at least two hours after a meal. Don't drink excessively just before you run either. Small sips over a longer period are preferable and it might help to avoid high sugar drinks too. Warming up gradually and easing yourself into your run could avoid triggering stitches, as could keeping your breathing relaxed and comfortable. If posture plays a role, then ensuring you have a strong core to maintain a good posture over a long distance might be the key for you. If you've recently started running and are plagued by stitches, then do persevere because they tend to become less frequent as you get fitter and your body adjusts to running.

Getting rid of a stitch

TRY THIS
AT HOME

Although side stitches can be incredibly painful, they aren't harmful and it's fine to keep running. There's little evidence to base a recommendation on, but here are some anecdotal things you can try to ease stitches while you're on the move:

- **Slow down** Taking your foot off the gas for a short time can be enough to help a stitch settle.

continued overleaf ▶

- **Deep breathing** Focus on filling your lungs properly (see page 59). Try counting and finding a regular breathing pattern.
- **Apply pressure** Pushing on the area where the stitch is can minimise movement and ease pain.
- **Stretch** Try stretching the affected side, so if your pain is under your ribs on the right-hand side, put your right hand on your head and bend to the left.
- **Touch your toes** Obviously you'll have to stop briefly to do this, but bending over forwards for a few breaths is a trick that works for many.
- **Time your foot strike** Some runners say that they can get rid of a stitch by exhaling as the foot on the opposite side to the stitch hits the ground. So for a right-sided stitch you need to breathe out as your left foot strikes the pavement.

Q I'm really windy when I run, burping and farting all over the place. Why is this?

A How much gas we each produce varies greatly and, whether it goes up or down, excess air needs to be expelled from the body somehow. It's normal to swallow some air when you run, especially if you're pushing yourself and gasping for breath, but particularly if you're trying to combine running and drinking. It's worth practising your 'on the move' fuelling and finding the bottle, cup or hydration pack mouthpiece that allows you to drink without gulping large quantities of air at the same time. Running itself may cause gas due to the jarring of the stomach and the faster transit of food through the gut. What you eat makes a difference too – some foods are more gaseous than others. Beans, lentils and cabbage are well known for making you trump, but so are other high-fibre foods such as fruit, bran and peas, as well as starchy foods and wholegrains. If windy runs are causing you problems, then it might be worth keeping a food diary to identify the culprits. Allow enough time for your food to digest before you run and eat slowly too, chewing food well to aid digestion and avoid swallowing air. Generally, there's no better time to let one loose than out in the fresh air, but spare a thought for those running close to you and, as a running friend of mine (with tricky bowels) says, 'Never trust a fart after 20 miles.'

Did you know?

The average person produces between 0.5 and 1.5 litres of flatus (gas) every 24 hours, and breaks wind between 10 and 20 times a day.

Q Running makes me need to poo. I have to plan my route around the local toilets.

A The dreaded runner's trots! You can be assured you are most definitely not alone. There are a few theories as to why vigorous exercise makes you need to poo, but there's no clear answer and it may be a combination of factors. It could be that jiggling your bowels around when you run irritates them or that, when you exercise, blood is diverted away from the bowel to the running muscles and the bowel doesn't appreciate this. We know that running helps ease constipation and the adrenalin released during exercise speeds up the time it takes for food to travel through the gut. If you have pre-race nerves, then there's even more adrenalin circulating and this effect can be heightened. It certainly explains why the motions are often loose and explosive, because a rapid transit time means there's less time for water reabsorption in the large intestine. There are numerous things you can try to prevent diarrhoea. It's usually a case of trial and error and being prepared. If you're new to running then don't be disheartened. Many runners find that as they get more experienced this issue bothers them less.

Resolving the runner's trots

If urgent trips to the toilet while you're running are ruining your fun, then try these tips to reduce the likelihood of you needing to divert to the nearest bush:

- **Help your digestion** Take your time when you eat. Sit down and chew your food properly. Smaller chunks will allow it to digest more easily. Allow enough time between eating and running. Everyone is different and digestion time also varies with what you eat, but an hour after a snack and two hours after a meal is a rough guide.
- **Choose your foods** If you struggle with the trots then keep a note of what you've eaten prior to running and the day before too. Food diaries can be really helpful to work out whether there's one food in particular which is causing problems. Spicy, rich or very fibrous foods are potential triggers.
- **Watch your drinks** Drinks can trigger the urgent need to do a poo too. Alcohol the night before running won't help your bowel, fruit juices can upset it and we know that caffeine is a stimulant, so while a quick pre-race espresso might help your performance, it might also speed up your guts.
- **Train your gut** You might notice that if you suddenly increase the frequency, intensity or distance of your running that your bowels object. This is often why those new to running have more problems than experienced runners. Making changes gradually allows your gut to adjust to the new levels of exertion.
- **Warm up** Wake your bowel up slowly with a good warm-up rather than suddenly diving straight into vigorous exercise. A slow walk speeding up to a brisk walk and then a jog might be sufficient to prevent suddenly needing the loo.

continued overleaf ▶

- **Fuel carefully** Over longer distances when you need race fuel you might find that highly concentrated or caffeine-containing sports supplements upset your gut. Experiment with normal food such as home-made energy balls, fruit loaf and bagels.
- **Calm down** If pre-race nerves are high, then your adrenalin levels will be surging and this might affect your bowel. Try to relax with deep breathing, distraction by friends or listening to music.
- **Be prepared** Arrive in plenty of time for races so you have time to queue for the loo at least once! Sometimes, however, it just happens out of the blue and despite all your tricks and practice the sudden urge is overwhelming. A tissue in your race belt weighs little and helps a lot if you have an unexpected bush stop or there's none left in the portaloo.

Q Is it OK to take an anti-diarrhoea tablet before a race?

You'll frequently see runners on online forums saying they take a medication to stop them having diarrhoea during a race. The most commonly used is loperamide, which slows down the movement of food though the bowel, allowing more time for water to be reabsorbed back into the bloodstream and thereby drying out the faeces. It also increases the tone of the anal sphincter (muscular ring keeping the anus closed) so it can help to reduce the urgency to pass a stool. Loperamide is used to control diarrhoea resulting from medical conditions. It isn't licensed for preventing exercise-induced diarrhoea. It can be an effective way to control the runner's trots if a dose is taken before running, but it's important to know what the side-effects or dangers are so you can decide if it's right for you.

Loperamide is designed to dry up faeces so you may end up constipated or with abdominal cramps. It can also make you feel sick, dizzy or give you a headache. All medications obviously have a risk of allergic reaction too. In 2017 there were reports of serious cardiac adverse reactions due to overdoses of loperamide, so never take more than the recommended dose. Although loperamide is available to buy over the counter, it may react badly with some prescribed medications so always check with the pharmacist. Don't take it for the first time on race day. Try it out beforehand and be aware it doesn't work for everyone. It's far better to look at your triggers and find other ways to control your bowels if you can. Never forget to see a doctor if you have blood in your stool or a persistent change in your bowel habit.

Q Will running help my irritable bowel syndrome?

A Irritable bowel syndrome (IBS) is a very common condition affecting around one in five people. Its causes are not fully understood. Symptoms include diarrhoea, constipation, bloating and abdominal pains, but indigestion, fatigue and headaches can be a feature too. Sometimes IBS can cause muscle pains, bladder symptoms and, for women, pain during sex. IBS can't be cured, but running is a great way to help manage it. It can keep constipation at bay, because it speeds up the passage of faeces through the bowel and it can help to reduce symptoms of bloating too.

The other way that running can help with IBS is by controlling mood and stress levels. We know that stress and tension in daily life can cause flare-ups of IBS. All runners know how much better they feel emotionally after a run so exercise can be used to stabilise mood, relieve stress and therefore manage IBS. There seems to be a close relationship between the brain and the gut. Certain antidepressant medications improve IBS symptoms even in people who aren't depressed. This may be because they reduce pain or have a direct effect on the nerve endings in the gut. When you run, your body releases natural versions of some of the chemicals that are in antidepressants, such as serotonin, a well-known feel-good chemical. So although we don't fully understand the mechanism, running can ease IBS through controlling stress, but it also seems to have a more direct action on the gut. However, it would be wrong not to mention that for some people with IBS running can trigger symptoms, especially if they suffer from excessive pre-race nerves or diarrhoea.

Real-life runners

I have IBS. I get a griping pain, a gurgling in my stomach and I *have* to go. It becomes all I can think about. For some reason it started affecting me 4km into runs. Thankfully a recent 10km race was a country route and I climbed over a gate and hid behind a hedge. Luckily I had tissues, but I pity the poor sheep! I was fine afterwards and could run again. I worked out the trigger was my breakfast and since swapping from Greek yoghurt and oats to a plain bagel it hasn't happened since. It certainly wasn't my finest hour and I was just glad it wasn't a city centre race!

Louise, parkrun director and cockerpoo owner (find me on the last page of the race results)

Q I've got food poisoning and can't get off the toilet today. I have a race at the weekend. Will I be OK to run?

A Bouts of food poisoning or other types of gastroenteritis can be as brief as 24 hours, but can last up to a week. Your digestive system is vigorously and efficiently ridding itself of its entire contents with vomiting or diarrhoea or, if you're unlucky, both at once. The biggest risk is dehydration. You can lose large amounts of fluid in vomit and loose stools. It can be hard to get sufficient intake when you're vomiting recurrently or liquids seem to be going straight through you. There's no doubt you will feel weak and drained after this illness and without sufficient recovery time you aren't going to be in good racing condition. Before you return to exercise you should have at least two full days of recovery when you can eat and drink normally without having diarrhoea or being sick. If you've had a short 24-hour bug and bounced back quickly then it may be reasonable to race following that recovery time, but don't expect a PB. Longer illnesses are going to need more time and recuperation, particularly if you're taking part in an endurance race. For now, concentrate on resting, sipping frequent, small amounts of fluid and make the call nearer the event.

Did you know?

The liver is the biggest solid organ in the body. It weighs approximately 1.5kg and it's the only organ that can regenerate itself.

Q Will drinking alcohol affect my running?

A The liver is part of the gastrointestinal system and has a huge number of roles in the body, including the breaking down and removal of alcohol from the bloodstream. As a rough guide, the body breaks down alcohol at a rate of one unit per hour. This means that it takes about two hours to break down a pint of beer and three hours for a large (250ml) glass of wine. How much alcohol affects you depends on a number of variables, including your gender (women break down alcohol more slowly than men), weight, metabolism and race (some Asians have an inherited deficiency in one of the enzymes which breaks down alcohol). A moderate alcohol intake is unlikely to have a significant negative influence on your general running, but you'd be hard pushed to claim it could have a positive one, apart from perhaps a glass of something to help you relax the night before a race. If you're looking for optimal performance, then these negative effects of alcohol might be enough to convince you to abstain:

- **Alcohol affects sleep** Even small amounts of alcohol can affect sleep quality. You may fall asleep more quickly, but you'll experience less restorative (REM) sleep and that will have a knock-on effect to your performance.

- **Alcohol can impair recovery** A few pints after a race is a nice way to celebrate, but a single, large amount of alcohol can affect skeletal muscle repair, impede hydration and affect glycogen synthesis as the body attempts to replenish its stores. How much is too much post-race has many variables, but 0.5g/kg of bodyweight is unlikely to have a significant effect on recovery. One unit contains 8g of alcohol so this works out at around two pints of beer (four units of alcohol) for a man weighing 70kg.

- **Alcohol contains empty calories** Alcohol is highly calorific (a 175ml glass of wine contains around 160 calories – equivalent to three ginger nut biscuits) but of no nutritional value. High-performance running requires nutrient-dense, high-quality food. Alcohol doesn't offer this and an excess can lead to weight gain.

- **Alcohol reduces immune function** Excessive long-term use and binge drinking can affect the body's ability to fight infection and heal injuries.

- **Alcohol causes dehydration** Alcohol is a diuretic, which means it increases the amount of urine produced and water is therefore lost from the body. Hydration is also important in temperature regulation so this may be disrupted too, further affecting performance.

- **Alcohol lowers blood sugar** Although blood sugar may rise initially, soon after a drink, once the liver gets busy removing the alcohol from the body, it neglects its role of regulating glucose. Insulin secretion is increased causing low glucose levels, which are not compatible with good sports performance.

Q Is it safe to run with a hangover?

A Obviously, the more alcohol you consumed and the later into the night you drank it, then the bigger the effect on your ability to exercise the next day. Whether you ate or not can also determine how good you feel. It's worth calculating how many units of alcohol you drank, because that will give you some idea as to whether it's likely to be out of your system. It takes approximately one hour for one unit of alcohol to be removed from the body. The negative effects of alcohol mean that there are a number of reasons why exercising with a hangover isn't a good idea. With poor sleep you'll be lacking in energy but may also find your co-ordination and balance are affected, which can increase your injury risk. You will be dehydrated from the alcohol and further dehydration from sweating through running will only add to this. When you're dehydrated you also have a faster pulse rate. Running will raise this further and put you at increased risk of developing abnormal heart rhythms such as atrial fibrillation. Your metabolism may not be in the best shape to endure a run either, especially if it's still trying to clear alcohol from your system and you need plenty of available glucose for running.

Whether a run is safe and whether it will make you feel better or worse really depends on how you feel. If you just have a bit of a thick head then your risks are low, but if you're dizzy, nauseated or have a racing heart then it makes sense to opt out or at least delay your run. Rehydrate as much as possible, make sure you're passing plenty of pale, yellow urine and take a drink with you when you run. Wait until your pulse rate has calmed down and also make sure you have eaten before you run to counteract the alcohol-induced low blood sugar levels. Just be sensible! Don't go if you don't feel up to it and if you do go take it very easy and see how you feel. Go home if you need to. There's always tomorrow.

Q I've just been diagnosed with coeliac disease. Will I have enough energy to run?

A If you have coeliac disease, your immune system attacks the healthy tissues of the gut when you eat gluten. In order for the tests for it to give an accurate answer, you need to have consumed some gluten in at least one meal a day for a minimum of six weeks before the test. Once you have the official diagnosis of coeliac disease you can begin a full gluten-free diet and you should find that your symptoms disappear quite quickly. Diarrhoea, abdominal pains and bloating will resolve and your energy levels will increase. There is no reason why you shouldn't run. In fact, you may notice an improvement in your performance as you begin to feel generally better in yourself. It's important to attend scheduled reviews with your doctor to check for any complications of coeliac disease and to see if you need any dietary supplements, such as iron, calcium or vitamin D. It's very helpful to see a dietician when you are diagnosed and at any point if you are struggling with symptoms again. Coeliac disease is not the same as gluten or wheat intolerance, allergy or sensitivity. It is an auto-immune condition where the lining of the small intestine becomes damaged, leading to abdominal symptoms and inadequate absorption of essential nutrients. It is a life-long condition which requires treatment and monitoring. When it is well-controlled – and the majority of people control it simply by following a gluten-free diet – then it shouldn't have any effect on your energy levels and ability to run.

Q I have Crohn's disease. I need surgery and will have a stoma and a bag. Will I be able to return to running?

A Absolutely yes! You'll need adequate time to recover from your surgery and a gradual return to core strengthening exercises and running, but a stoma needn't stop you. Search online for lots of inspiring stories and blogs from people running with stomas and ostomy bags (a stoma is an opening surgically created in the abdomen so that waste can leave the body and an ostomy bag is what the waste is collected in). It might take some trial and error to find the right bag for you to run with and similarly the best way to secure your bag. There are belts and specially designed wraps, as well as high-waisted running leggings to ensure your bag is snug and you feel confident. Other runners probably won't be able to tell you have a bag, but you can choose loose-fitting tops if you're self-conscious. Getting your hydration and fuelling right can take a bit of practice. It's extremely unlikely your bag will burst, but reducing gas and wind (see page 73) will minimise this risk if you are concerned.

Q I have a family history of bowel cancer. Will running reduce my risk?

A In fact, 95 per cent of bowel cancers are not due to an inherited gene. If your affected relative is first degree (mother, father or sibling) and had their cancer diagnosed before they were 50, there might be a genetic cause. Similarly, if your first degree relative was older, but had a first degree relative who was affected, then this may be significant. If you're concerned about the likelihood of inherited cancer, then speak to your GP. There is strong evidence that regular exercise can reduce the risk of developing bowel cancer by 25 to 50 per cent. This is a striking figure. Exercise speeds up the passage of faeces through the gut and reduces the amount of contact time that any carcinogens (cancer forming substances) have with the bowel wall. Exercise also causes the release of natural killer cells and lowers inflammation levels in the body, both of which help to reduce cancer risk (see page 207). So making a commitment to running regularly is a powerful way to lower your risk of this common condition, whether you have a family history of it or not.

Q I've got piles which hurt and bleed. Has running caused this and what can I do?

A Running may have caused or worsened your piles (haemorrhoids) if you've been spending many hours running long distances. Both vigorous activity and being on your feet for a long time increase pressure on the blood vessels in the rectum. Piles are essentially swollen veins and fleshy tissue which form small lumps, either inside or just outside your anus. There are many causes of piles, other than endurance running. Child birth, straining on the toilet and sitting for long periods of time are frequently to blame. You may also have a genetic tendency to develop them. It's crucial to make sure you are well-hydrated and avoid constipation. Exercise prevents constipation, but be sure to drink plenty of fluids after a run to fully rehydrate. A diet rich in fibre will help smooth the transit of stools through your gut. Piles usually shrink and disappear on their own, but speak to your pharmacist about creams you can use to soothe them and reduce any itching in the meantime. Apply a product like Sudocrem to help protect the delicate piles from sweat and chafing while you run, and make sure you clean and dry the area thoroughly after running. Blood from the back passage can be due to other more serious causes so don't rely on self-diagnosis and see your GP. Don't feel embarrassed to get it checked out – they've seen it all before.

Did you know?

The time it takes food to go from entering your mouth to passing out of your anus as waste is called 'transit time'. Transit time varies hugely between individuals and is influenced by what foods and fluids have been consumed, but is approximately 24 to 72 hours. Most of this time is spent in the large bowel. Women have a longer bowel transit time than men and children have a shorter one than adults.

TOP TIPS FOR A HEALTHY RUNNER'S GUTS

- Keep a food diary and use trial and error to help solve gut issues.
- Drink plenty of fluid and rehydrate properly after runs to avoid constipation.
- Assist your digestion by avoiding over eating or eating in a rush. Chew your food properly and allow enough time between eating and running.
- See your doctor if you have a persistent change in your bowel habit or any blood loss from your back passage.
- Eat a healthy varied diet with plenty of whole grain fibre (unless you have IBS and find whole grains aggravate it).
- Look after your gut microbiome. Keep the good bacteria in your gut happy by eating plenty of plant-based foods and live yoghurts, and avoiding excess alcohol.
- Manage your stress levels.
- Don't smoke. It increases your risk of acid reflux and stomach cancer.

FURTHER HELP AND ADVICE

Coeliac UK: www.coeliac.org.uk

Crohn's and Colitis UK: www.crohnsandcolitis.org.uk

The IBS Network: www.theibsnetwork.org

NHS IBS diet video guide: www.nhs.uk/conditions/irritable-bowel-syndrome-ibs/ibs-diet-video-guide/

Drinkaware: www.drinkaware.co.uk

Macmillan Cancer Support www.macmillan.org.uk

CHAPTER 5

....

THE URINARY SYSTEM

As runners, we're repeatedly told how important it is for us to stay hydrated, so the urinary system, where water is both retained and lost from the body, is crucial for us. Understanding how that system works and being aware of potential problems will help us to run safely and healthily. So whether it's a leaky bladder, a troublesome prostate or concerns about kidney damage, this chapter has it covered. Grab a big drink of water and read on!

The urinary system includes your kidneys, bladder, ureters (tubes from kidney to bladder) and urethra (tube from bladder to the outside). Its main functions are to control the fluid balance of the body and to produce urine to remove toxins.

Around 150 litres of blood pass through your kidneys each day. Most people have two kidneys but it's possible to live normally and healthily with just one. You may have heard the kidneys' role described as 'cleaning the blood' and this paints a perfect picture. Kidneys contain about a million nephrons. These are filtering units which sort through the blood, taking out the bad bits and keeping the good. The way they do this is mind-blowingly clever. Blood arrives at the kidneys in the renal artery. The pressure in this artery is pretty high and the blood is pushed forcefully through the first part of the nephron, called the glomerulus. This is a knot of thin-walled blood vessels that act as a

The Urinary System

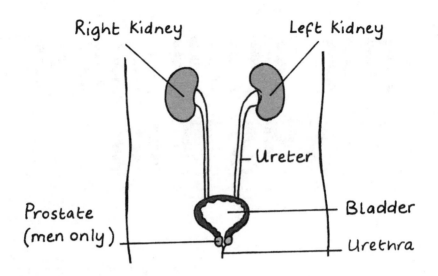

Right Kidney

Left Kidney

Ureter

Prostate
(men only)

Bladder

Urethra

The Nephron

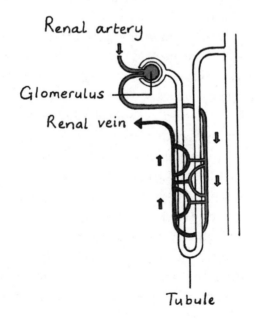

Renal artery

Glomerulus

Renal vein

Tubule

sieve. Big molecules such as blood cells and proteins remain in the blood while smaller ones such as urea (a waste product), water and ions like sodium slip through the sieve and into the kidney tubule to form urine. However, not all the small molecules are bad, so the kidney needs to selectively take back the ones it needs. The kidney tubule is long and runs close to the blood vessels so water, glucose and other nutrients can be reabsorbed back into the blood, ensuring only unwanted waste makes it to the urine.

Kidneys also have an important role in maintaining blood pressure. They detect pressure, fluid and body salt levels and can secrete a substance called renin, which triggers a system called the renin-angiotensin system. If blood pressure is falling then angiotensin will constrict the blood vessels, to increase pressure and also trigger release of a hormone called aldosterone from the adrenal glands, which are located just above each kidney. Aldosterone messages the kidneys to reabsorb more sodium and water from its tubules, which increases the blood volume and restores the balance again. If blood pressure is too high then the blood vessels are dilated and the kidneys take back less sodium and water to reduce the blood volume and pressure.

The ureters transport urine from the kidneys to the bladder where it's stored until you want to have a wee. The bladder is actually a muscular bag which can expand and then shrink back down again. It can hold about 500mls of urine and when it's getting stretched, it sends messages to your brain that it would be a good idea to find a toilet. When the time is right, the bladder muscle (called the detrusor muscle) contracts, forcing the urine out. At the same time, the sphincters and pelvic floor muscles, which keep urine in, relax and allow the urine to flow.

It's a complex system with many functions which are crucial to us as runners. Let's look at some questions related to the urinary system to further help us understand how it all works and to make sure we can run healthily.

Q I know that hydration is important for runners, but how much should I drink when I run?

A How much fluid you need when running depends on many variables, including your weight, the air temperature, your fitness, how much you sweat, your intensity and duration of exercise, what you've eaten... the list goes on and on. If you want to get very technical about it then you can follow the steps below to see how much fluid you've lost during a run. You do need to remember that there will be day-to-day variation so you can't assume this amount is what you need every time. It's just a guide. The simple answer is to just be directed by your thirst. You may have heard of the concept that if you're thirsty you're already dehydrated, but your thirst mechanism is well-designed and very sensitive. It will let you know when taking on water would be a good idea and it will tell you well ahead of time. You just need to tune into it. If you've had a drink before you exercise then you might not need one at all during activity unless it's a very hot day, your effort level is intense or you're running for over an hour. There are plenty of experienced runners doing ten-mile weekend runs without drinking while they're on the move. We can sometimes get too hung up on the whole water issue. It's sensible to take water with you on longer runs and drink to thirst. What you drink is important too, because replacing fluids lost through running means replacing salts as well as water.

Did you know?

Sweating is our body's way of cooling us down. Heat is lost when sweat evaporates from our skin. We have millions of sweat glands in our skin with more in areas such as our armpits, forehead and palms. Sweat contains mostly water, but also lactic acid and urea. Minerals such as sodium, potassium, calcium and magnesium are lost in sweat, as are tiny amounts of trace metals such as iron, copper and zinc.

Q What is hyponatraemia and how can I avoid it?

A Hyponatraemia means low blood sodium levels. Sodium is a mineral which the body's nerves and muscles need to function properly, but it also plays a crucial role in fluid balance in the body. Have you heard of osmosis, the process by which water is drawn across a membrane from a less concentrated solution to a more concentrated one? The kidney uses sodium to enable osmosis. Ions such as sodium are initially filtered out of the blood by the kidney, and into the tubule, to make urine. The kidney then selectively reabsorbs sodium back into the blood. By doing this it increases the concentration of sodium in the blood and water is then drawn in too. By moving sodium and regulating blood concentration, the kidney can move water back into the system to maintain fluid balance and blood pressure. If you ingest excess salt, then high sodium levels can mean that more water is drawn into your bloodstream and high blood pressure can result.

Sweat contains large amounts of sodium, so over a run of marathon distance or longer, you can lose significant amounts. At the same time, ingesting large quantities of water will literally dilute your blood. The result can be hyponatraemia – potentially dangerous low sodium levels, where cells begin to swell with water and malfunction. Hyponatraemia can present as weakness, confusion, cramps, nausea, headaches and, in severe cases, seizures and even death. This is why long-distance runners need to pay attention to their hydration and not drink large quantities of water at every drink station. Drinking to thirst is better and also making sure that some of what is consumed contains electrolytes (minerals), which include sodium. You can use specifically designed sports rehydration drinks or you can make your own using fruit squash and a pinch of salt. Sodium can also be replaced through eating salty foods such as pretzels or taking salt tablets. The longer and hotter the race, the bigger the risk. Being aware of the potential of hyponatraemia is important, but at the same time don't limit your fluid intake because you are scared of it, because you'll be at risk of harmful dehydration instead! Use your common sense, adapt to race conditions and practise your fuelling to minimise your risks.

Running hydration

TRY THIS AT HOME

If you're concerned about your hydration or simply curious about how much fluid you're losing during a run, then you can try this simple test. This will give you a good idea about how much you sweat, but don't forget that you lose fluid through your breathing and panting too.

1. Immediately before you run, weigh yourself naked.
2. Go for a run (dressed!) – a one-hour run is recommended.
3. After your run, strip naked again, towel dry off any sweat and weigh yourself.
4. Subtract your after-run weight from your pre-run weight and convert this to millilitres, e.g. 70kg–69kg = 1kg and 1kg = 1000mls.
5. If you have had a drink during your run, then add it to this total, e.g. 1000mls + 250mls = 1250mls.
6. This total is your fluid loss over the hour of running – 1250mls or 1.25 litres per hour.

You don't need to arrive home in perfect fluid balance. This will just give you an idea how much you need to replace after you've run and help you decide how much to drink while you're on the move. Remember, it is only a guide and will vary according to how hot or cold the weather is, how intense your session was and other daily variables. If you need to wee or poo then you'll have to do it before the pre-run weighing or after the post-run weighing, otherwise you'll be losing body fluids that haven't been measured.

Q Can running a marathon cause kidney damage?

A Learning about the hard work the kidneys have to do to maintain fluid balance, it may make you wonder whether running marathons, where hydration can be pushed to its limits, could actually harm the kidneys. Previous studies have shown that up to 85 per cent of ultramarathon runners have some degree of temporary kidney damage at the end of a race. But what about marathons? A small study of 22 marathon runners (41 per cent men), in the 2015 Hartford Marathon in the USA, found evidence of kidney damage with 73 per cent of the runners tested immediately after the marathon showing changes that indicated injury to the tubules of the kidney. Further tests taken 24 hours later showed some improvement, but not complete resolution of these changes. A different study of 167 amateur runners, between age 39 and 61, at the Berlin marathon showed that abnormalities in kidney function induced by running all returned to normal within two weeks after a marathon. What we don't know is what happens beyond that. Could years of repeated acute episodes of stress on the kidneys affect their future function? Or is the opposite true – that these periods of hardship only act to strengthen and maximise the response of the kidney to injury and are in fact protective? We aren't even sure exactly what it is about marathon running that causes damage to the kidneys. It's perhaps a lack of blood flow to the kidneys, dehydration, damage from muscle breakdown or a rise in core body temperature – it may well be a combination of all four.

There are blood tests that are used to check for chronic kidney disease (CKD), which is essentially 'wear and tear' on the kidneys, and these are frequently carried out on people with medical conditions such as diabetes and high blood pressure. It would be interesting to know if life-long endurance runners have a higher or lower incidence of CKD, but runners are healthier, less likely to have medical conditions or see the doctor for routine tests, so it would be hard to prove. What we can be sure of is that regular exercise helps to lower our risk of high blood pressure and type 2 diabetes, both important causes of kidney disease. We can look after our kidneys by keeping hydrated, respecting hot weather running and training sensibly. So far there isn't convincing evidence that running marathons damages your kidneys in the long term.

Did you know?

Each kidney measures 10 to 15 centimetres long and weighs around 160 grams which is equivalent to the weight of three tennis balls.

Q Is it safe to use anti-inflammatories when you run? I've heard it can damage the kidneys.

A Non-Steroidal Anti-Inflammatories (NSAIDs) are a family of drugs which include ibuprofen, diclofenac and naproxen. Ibuprofen can be bought over the counter in the UK and is widely used by runners, because it gives effective relief for musculoskeletal pain. It's not uncommon for runners to take ibuprofen before a long run in anticipation of pain, particularly when they want to perform well in a race or when they are running with an injury. We know that long-term use of NSAIDs can cause health problems, including kidney damage, high blood pressure, heart attacks and gastrointestinal ulcers, but will a single dose before an endurance run pose any risk? Anecdotally up to 75 per cent of ultramarathon runners take ibuprofen before racing so this population is ideal for identifying any potential harm to kidneys. A study published in 2017 gave either ibuprofen or a placebo to 89 runners, to take every four hours during their 50-mile run. Kidney function was tested immediately on finishing the race and 39 of the 89 runners had signs of acute kidney injury at the end of their race. The risk was 18 per cent higher in those that took ibuprofen. For every five runners who took ibuprofen there was one extra case of kidney damage. From this we can conclude that taking ibuprofen during an endurance race increased the risk of kidney damage in this population.

NSAIDs reduce the amount of blood flow in the kidneys and inhibit the formation of prostaglandins, which usually cause dilation of the blood vessels and increased filtration rates in the kidney. If we add the negative effect of dehydration too then we can begin to see why taking ibuprofen during endurance runs is not a risk-free option.

Q The nurse said there was blood in my urine when he did a dip test during a health check. Could this be related to running?

A dip stick urine test will detect blood in the urine that is not visible to the naked eye. We call this microscopic haematuria (blood which you can actually see in the urine is called macroscopic haematuria). Microscopic haematuria can happen for a number of reasons, including infection, prostate enlargement and bladder or kidney stones. It can also be due to kidney damage and bladder cancer, so it is an important sign. Sometimes the blood is simply coming from sore or cracked skin near the urethra or from contamination by menstrual blood in women. Strenuous exercise can cause blood to leak into the urine. This can be due to the bladder walls hitting against each other during running and blood coming from the resultant 'bruise'. If the kidney's nephron or cleaning function is impaired, it may also be due to red blood cells being pushed through the glomerulus, the knot of blood vessels that acts as a sieve (see page 88). This reduced nephron function may be as a result of decreased blood flow to the kidney when blood is diverted to skeletal muscles during exercise. It seems to be the intensity of exercise which is important and not just the distance run.

So, we are left with a conundrum. Exercise-induced microscopic haematuria not due to an underlying sinister cause will resolve and doesn't need any treatment, but recurrently having blood in your urine requires investigation to rule out treatable and significant medical conditions. You will definitely need to have at least one more urine test to determine the next steps. Your nurse or doctor may suggest you avoid strenuous exercise for 24 hours before this. They will need to take the rest of your medical history and the likelihood of other medical conditions causing the haematuria into account before deciding on the best course of action. If your microscopic haematuria is present on multiple dip stick tests, then you will need to have some investigations to look for the cause before assuming it is exercise-related. If it turns out to be purely exercise-related, then it's worth discussing with your doctor whether you need to take iron supplements to counteract this silent blood loss (see page 38).

Real-life runners

When I found blood in my urine, I suspected it was either an infection or most likely haematuria from running. However, I decided to get a professional opinion and I am glad I did as it turns out it I actually had prostate cancer. My advice is always seek a medical opinion as you never know what it could be.

Richard Hayes, runner, LEGO consultant and coffee lover

Q My friend peed blood after an ultra. Is this normal or should he be worried?

A Blood might be bright red and have some small clots in it or it might be diluted in the urine, turning it pink in colour. The potential causes are the same as those for microscopic haematuria, but the blood loss is heavier and is usually most pronounced on the first wee after a run. It tends to occur after distances of 10km or more and is usually painless. The same conundrum of when and how much to investigate arises, but ultimately blood in the urine must always be investigated so testing is important.

It's also important to know that urine can turn a red colour for reasons other than red blood cells being present. Eating dark red foods such as beetroot can result in red urine which is easily mistaken for blood loss. It can also be due to myoglobinuria – myoglobin is a protein found in skeletal muscle. When muscles are damaged and break down (a process called rhabdomyolysis), myoglobin is released and the kidneys filter it out and excrete it in urine, because high levels can be toxic to the kidneys. Myoglobin turns the urine a red/brown colour, a bit like cola, which can be mistaken for blood. Myoglobinuria and rhabdomyolysis can occur in runners after ultramarathons. It usually resolves with time and adequate fluid intake, but there are situations where this may be dangerous and the risk of kidney failure increases. These include dehydration, extreme heat, taking NSAIDs, and running with or soon after a viral or bacterial infection. If you have cola-coloured urine after an endurance race you should seek an urgent medical assessment.

Did you know?

Adults produce about 1.5 litres of urine every 24 hours, but anywhere between 0.5 and 2.5 litres can be normal, depending on your size and how much fluid you've drunk.

Q Why do I leak urine when I run and what can I do about it?

A Around a third of women report leaking urine when they run so you are not alone. The actual figure may be much higher than that, because women find it embarrassing and don't tell anyone. This type of leaking is called stress incontinence. Running is basically repetitive jumping – you have two feet off the ground at one time and the impact of returning to the ground causes an increased pressure inside the pelvis. Ordinarily the pelvic floor muscles would be able to cope with this, but if these muscles are weak then they're unable to support the bladder enough to prevent urine leaking out. Being pregnant and giving birth weakens the pelvic floor, particularly if the baby was big or the delivery difficult. Pelvic floor muscles can also be weakened by the falling oestrogen levels of the menopause – as many as half of women over 50 experience some urinary leaking. Straining with constipation, recurrent coughing and being overweight can all stress and damage the pelvic floor muscles.

The first thing to do is to realise that while stress incontinence is common, it's not normal. You don't need to put up with wet running shorts and treatment is available. Ideally you should have an assessment by a women's health physiotherapist. They are trained to examine and advise you. You can ask your GP to refer you or, if you have the means, you can make a private appointment. Your individual situation will be assessed and you will be given a programme of exercises to help restore your continence. This will involve pelvic floor exercises, but it will also include other specific exercises to correct any muscular imbalances that may be adding to the problem, for example weak glute muscles. The physiotherapist may also use a range of devices to help you identify and strengthen your pelvic floor muscles, such as electrical stimulation probes and vaginal exercisers. With perseverance and hard work, over 60 per cent of women find the treatment successful, but it can take months so don't give up. As the issue of urinary incontinence becomes less taboo and awareness of the problems increases, there is more work being done to offer solutions to women, including pessaries to insert during exercise and sports shorts designed by a female engineer which mimic the structure and support of the pelvic floor muscles.

Real-life runners

I started running aged 56. It was when I started entering events and trying to run hard down hills that I found I was leaking a bit of urine. My GP recommended an app for pelvic floor exercises. This was great and along with more advanced exercises from a specialist physiotherapist, the problem was solved.

Margaret, runner, explorer and triathlete

Did you know?

Pelvic floor muscle exercises are also called Kegels, after the American gynaecologist Arnold Kegel. In the 1950s he invented a device called the Kegel perineometer to measure the strength of pelvic floor muscle contractions. He used this alongside Kegel exercises to help treat urinary incontinence.

Q Should runners do pelvic floor exercises and do men need to do them too?

A Yes and yes! The pelvic floor is a sling of muscles that runs from your pubic bone at the front to your coccyx (sitting bone) at the back. It supports your pelvic organs, including your bladder, bowel and the uterus in women. It has an important role in helping you stay continent, and weak pelvic floor muscles can result in both urinary and faecal incontinence. Weakness can result from excess pressure on the muscles such as strain from coughing, constipation, heavy lifting or being overweight. In women, childbirth and falling oestrogen levels of the menopause can weaken it too. You can strengthen the pelvic floor muscles with specific exercises and this will improve symptoms of incontinence in the majority of sufferers. The pelvic floor muscles are also involved with erectile function and having a strong pelvic floor might help you maintain an erection, prevent premature ejaculation and result in stronger orgasms. They're important for everyone, male or female, and particularly important for those doing high impact sports such as running.

Pelvic floor exercises

TRY THIS AT HOME

Be warned: identifying and controlling your pelvic floor muscles can take time and practice. With perseverance and regular practice you can expect to see an improvement in any continence problems within three months.

Identify the muscles The pelvic floor muscles loop around both your urethra (water works tube) and your anus. Imagine you are in a very important meeting where breaking wind is completely inappropriate. Try to squeeze the muscles that would keep the wind in. These are the muscles around your anus that you need to work. When you are next passing urine, try to stop mid-flow and feel how the muscles contract. These are the muscles around your urethra that you need to work. Men should see their scrotum lift upwards and their penis nod downwards a little. Don't stop mid-flow regularly, only to help you find the correct muscles to squeeze. Squeezing these front and back muscles and drawing them up together and towards each other is what you need to do during the following pelvic floor exercises.

Work the muscles You can do these exercises sitting down (easiest way to start), standing or lying, anywhere at any time. No one will know you are doing them. Remember, you shouldn't be squeezing your bottom, raising your eyebrows or holding your breath while you do them. The pelvic floor has both fast- and slow-twitch muscle fibres and you need to work them both.

continued overleaf ▶

1. Take a deep breath in, ensuring you fill your belly (see page 59). Your pelvic floor will relax when you do this.
2. As you slowly exhale, work the fast-twitch fibres by performing five short, sharp squeezes of the pelvic floor muscles.
3. Repeat this five times making sure you fully relax your pelvic floor while you inhale.
4. Now move on to the slow-twitch fibres. Take a deep breath in. Exhale slowly and gradually draw the front and back pelvic floor muscles upwards and together. Imagine an elevator travelling up the floors. As you get stronger you will be able to hold onto the slow squeeze for your entire exhalation. Aim for five to 10 seconds.
5. Repeat this five times, slowly relaxing your pelvic floor muscles back to complete rest while you breathe in.

Do these exercises three times a day for the rest of your life. You may only feel a flicker of movement when you first start these exercises, but don't worry. They will get stronger with regular practice. Concentrating fully on the muscles will help you properly connect with them. If you can't identify them, they are too weak to squeeze or aren't getting stronger with practice, then see your GP.

Q Is it safe to run with a vaginal prolapse?

A In women, the bladder, bowel or uterus can sometimes drop down from their normal position and give a sensation of dragging or aching in the vagina, and sometimes a bulge or lump can appear. The usual cause is weak pelvic floor muscles that aren't giving these organs the structural support they need. The symptoms experienced depend on which organs are prolapsing. If it's the bladder that's dropping down, then it's called a cystocele and you may experience urinary incontinence, or need to pass urine frequently and urgently. You may also find that you don't empty your bladder properly or that the flow of urine is blocked in some way. If it's the bowel that's dropping down, then it's called a recotocele, which can make passing faeces difficult. Symptoms are usually worse when you have been on your feet for a while and gravity has been at work.

Having a vaginal prolapse indicates that there is dysfunction of your pelvic floor and you shouldn't add extra pressure to it by running. The high impact nature of running may make your prolapse worse. You need to be assessed and treated before you run again. Mild prolapses can usually be resolved with pelvic floor exercises. More severe prolapses may require insertion of a pessary (plastic ring or shelf) to supplement the pelvic floor muscles or possible surgery. Keeping to a healthy weight, avoiding constipation and delegating heavy lifting can help stop prolapses worsening too.

Q Running seems to help most health conditions. Can it help prostate problems?

A The prostate is a small gland that sits just below the bladder in men. It makes fluid which forms part of semen, and during ejaculation the muscles of the prostate contract and push the fluid out into the urethra to carry and nourish the sperm. The three most common types of prostate problem are prostatitis (inflammation, often due to infection), benign prostatic hypertrophy (BPH), where the prostate is enlarged, and prostate cancer. All three can cause prostate symptoms which include needing to pass urine frequently, difficulty initiating the stream of urine, a weak stream of urine and dribbling urine after finishing.

Physical activity is unlikely to have any bearing on prostatitis, although men with a chronic (greater than six months' duration) prostatitis may find that exercise helps to reduce symptoms and increase wellbeing in what can be a challenging condition to control. Several studies, however, have examined the relationship between exercise and BPH. There have been conflicting results, with some showing that low intensity exercise might reduce the risk of BPH more than vigorous exercise and others showing that vigorous exercise might actually increase the risk of BPH. One study done in 2008 used data from the National Runners' Health Study which included over 28,000 men. It relied on self-reporting of diagnosis and running distances but it concluded that exercise, regardless of the BMI, diet or 10km pace of the runner, may lower the risk of BPH and that potentially longer distances mean larger reductions. A Cochrane review (a systematic review of primary health research) in 2019 examined all relevant studies done to determine whether exercise could be used as a first-line treatment for the symptoms of BPH. Unfortunately, they found such low-quality evidence they were unable to draw any conclusions, so further research is most definitely needed.

The jury is also still out on exactly whether and by how much exercise might reduce the risk of prostate cancer. So far, it is pointing to yes – vigorous exercise may be most effective and the biggest risk reduction is in aggressive prostate cancer (see page 207).

Did you know?

The average number of times people pass urine in 24 hours is six or seven.

Q My bladder is so sensitive I have to visit the portaloo many times before a race and stop during runs. What can I do about it?

A Sometimes it isn't a leaky bladder that causes problems, it's an overactive one that doesn't seem to hold much, always needs to empty and can make you live in fear that if you don't go to the toilet you might wet yourself. Both men and women can suffer from an overactive bladder (OAB). Around 15 per cent of men have the condition and it is under-recognised and often under-treated in men because of their hesitancy to seek help. It's particularly common in post-menopausal women where low oestrogen levels can lead to bladder muscle irritability and atrophy (thinning) and irritation of the tissues around the urethra and vagina resulting in increased urinary frequency.

Here are some things that might help:

- **Stay calm** In a race situation, nerves will almost certainly add to the problem, so try to relax and distract yourself.
- **Avoid irritants** OAB can be made worse by caffeine and alcohol, so steer clear of these.
- **Drink plenty** This may sound counter-intuitive, but simply reducing what you drink to avoid needing to go the toilet will just make urine more concentrated and irritating, and may harm your running performance.
- **Train your bladder** You may need to do this with professional help, but it is possible to retrain your bladder by gradually leaving longer and longer gaps between going to the toilet, aiming for every four hours. When you feel you need to go then change what you're doing, distract yourself or do some pelvic floor exercises.
- **See your GP** If this is a new symptom for you then you may need to have some tests to look for an underlying cause such as urinary tract infection, diabetes, bladder or prostate problems. Once a diagnosis of OAB has been made then there are medications that can be used to relax the bladder. They aren't without their side-effects, but can be very helpful for some people. Women with vaginal atrophy can use an oestrogen cream to plump up the thinned tissues and relieve symptoms. Bladder botox injections aren't available everywhere, but can provide short-term, effective relief. In extreme circumstances, nerve stimulation and bladder surgery may be offered.

Collecting a urine sample

TRY THIS AT HOME

Ever had a urine pot thrust into your hand at the doctors with advice to provide a sample? Here's the best way to collect urine and minimise the risk of it being contaminated, which can mean a useless result.

1. Wash your hands. If you're at home then wash your genital area too.
2. Wrap some toilet paper around the outside of the specimen pot, particularly if you're a woman as aiming your stream of urine is tricky.
3. Unscrew the lid of the pot. Be careful not to touch the inside to keep it sterile.
4. Women should sit on the toilet with their legs apart and use one hand to hold back the labia so urine can flow out with minimal contact with the skin. Men can retract the foreskin for the same reason.
5. Start to pass urine, but don't collect the first bit. A mid-stream sample is best if the sample is looking for possible infection.
6. Pop the pot under the stream of urine and collect your sample.
7. Screw the lid back on and throw away the tissue you wrapped around the outside.
8. Wash your hands.
9. Label the container if it hasn't already been done for you.

Q I run a lot and I get a lot of cystitis. Is there a link?

A Cystitis means inflammation of the bladder and it can sometimes be caused by infection, but often by irritation too. Symptoms include needing to wee frequently, stinging and burning when you pass urine, and bladder pain. It's much more common in women than men and there's often a trigger, such as having sex or going swimming. There may be a link with running for you. The urethra brings urine from the bladder to the outside and the urethral opening can be quite delicate. Rubbing underwear, shorts or tights can irritate this area and cause superficial pain, and stinging or burning when you wee. To reduce this, apply some lubricant or baby's nappy cream to the area before you run. It will act as a barrier and protect the delicate tissues. Runners often wash frequently and using soaps, bubble baths and shower gels can trigger cystitis. Taking a shower rather than a bath and avoiding using perfumed products will help to reduce the risk – plain water is fine for cleaning your genitals.

Another way running could be linked to your cystitis is by irritation of the bladder lining. The action of running and the jolting it causes may lead to the bladder walls hitting each other, which can inflame them. Similarly, if you don't hydrate enough then concentrated urine might irritate the bladder lining too. This shows how important it is to hydrate well, especially in the hours after you run. Of course, cystitis is common and yours may be unrelated to running. If you are having frequent bouts, then do see your GP to discuss and take a urine sample with you to the appointment. This is particularly important if you are male as urine infections are much less common and the threshold for investigation is lower.

Q Can I exercise with a urine infection?

A The severity of a urinary tract infection (UTI) can vary hugely. It can make you feel very unwell, especially if your kidneys are involved. In this situation you're likely to have a high temperature, nausea or vomiting and back pain. Running is clearly not a good idea and you should rest and recover. Similarly, if you have blood in your urine, stinging when you pee or abdominal pain, then give running a miss. If on the other hand you've just had a couple of extra trips to the toilet and it was a bit uncomfortable, but you otherwise feel fine, then going for a run probably isn't going to do you any harm. Do make sure you drink plenty of water, though, because concentrated urine is only going to make things worse. Urine infections are usually treated with antibiotics, so see your GP if mild symptoms aren't settling after a couple of days, you feel unwell or your symptoms are more severe.

TOP TIPS FOR A HEALTHY RUNNER'S URINARY SYSTEM

- Hydrate yourself before, during (if necessary) and after your runs.
- Replace electrolytes lost through sweat, especially on long runs (see page 91).
- Respect the weather conditions and adapt your expectations, pace and hydration in hot weather.
- Don't use anti-inflammatory medications for pain relief during long runs and races.
- Get your blood pressure checked at least every five years or more often if there's a medical need. High blood pressure can damage the kidneys.
- Eat a healthy diet and drink plenty of fluid to avoid constipation, which can affect bladder function.
- Do regular pelvic floor exercises.
- Don't suffer in silence and seek help if you experience urinary or faecal incontinence.
- If you have given birth then make a gradual, planned return to running after strengthening your pelvic floor muscles (see page 100).

FURTHER HELP AND ADVICE

Kidney Care UK: www.kidneycareuk.org

The National Kidney Foundation: www.kidney.org

Prostate Cancer UK: www.prostatecanceruk.org

Bladder and Bowel Community: www.bladderandbowel.org

Bladder and Bowel UK: www.bbuk.org.uk

Disability UK: www.disabilityrightsuk.org

Incontinence UK: www.incontinence.co.uk

SqueezyApp pelvic floor exercises: www.squeezyapp.com

Engineered sportswear for women: EVB Sport www.evbsport.com

CHAPTER 6

....

THE REPRODUCTIVE SYSTEM

L et's move on down to the reproductive system. You might not immediately think that this system is terribly relevant to running, but once you start considering it you'll soon see it is! It can cause huge problems, especially for women, but running also offers many benefits for the reproductive system in terms of physical, mental and sexual health. This information is intentionally not split into separate men's and women's sections, because it's important we have an insight and understanding into the barriers all our running friends face. Let's quickly recap the basic anatomy of both the male and female reproductive systems so we're clear on exactly what lies where.

The male reproductive system includes the penis, the contents of the scrotum, the prostate and seminal vesicles (the glands that make the fluid for semen). We've already covered the prostate (see page 102) so here we'll just be dealing with the crown jewels. Inside the scrotum you'll find two testicles, each with an epididymis and a vas deferens. Sperm is made in the testicle and stored in the epididymis until ejaculation, when it travels along the vas deferens, mixes with fluid from the prostate and seminal vesicles, and leaves as semen via

The Male Reproductive System

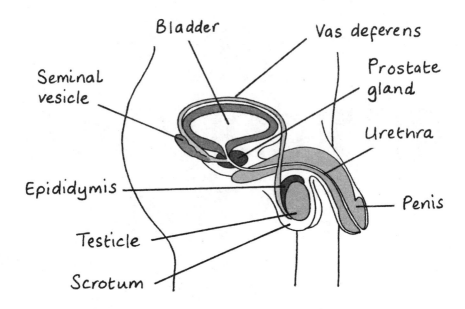

the urethra in the penis. The testicles also make hormones, including testosterone, the main male hormone. Testosterone has many roles in the body other than sperm production, including regulating sex drive, controlling muscle, bone and fat metabolism, and prompting red blood cell production. Testosterone can also influence mood and behaviour.

The Female Reproductive System

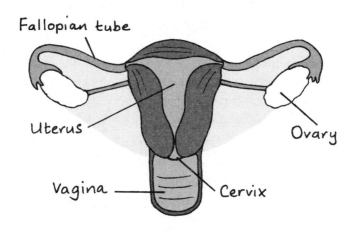

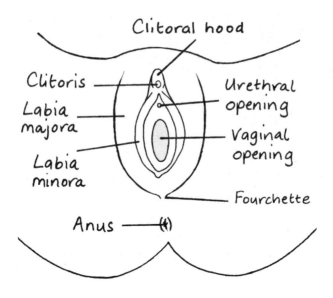

The female reproductive system includes the uterus, ovaries, fallopian tubes, cervix, vagina and vulva. The ovaries make the main female hormones, progesterone and oestrogen. They also make small amounts of testosterone. The two ovaries take it in turns to release an egg each month. This is called ovulation. The egg travels along the fallopian tube and, if it meets a sperm, it can become fertilised, nestle into the wall of the uterus and result in a pregnancy. If it's not fertilised by a sperm then the lining of the uterus, which has been bulked up for possible pregnancy, is shed in a monthly bleed. The menstrual blood passes through the cervix (neck of the womb) and into the vagina. The vagina opens to the outside in the vulva. Many people (men and women) get the terminology wrong. The vulva is not the vagina. The vulva is the whole area inside the lips, also called the labia majora, and includes the inner lips (labia minora), the clitoris, the urethral (water works) opening and the vaginal opening. More information on all aspects of the female reproductive system, including menstruation, periods, pregnancy and menopause, is covered in my previous book, *Sorted: The Active Woman's Guide to Health*.

Problems and questions related to these systems crop up all the time, so let's dive in and consider them. We'll start with sex and move onto fertility, periods, pregnancy and beyond.

Q Will sex the night before a race help my performance or am I better to abstain?

A In the past there has been a view that having sex before a sporting fixture could decrease performance, and that a degree of sexual frustration would lead to a more aggressive, competitive and successful performance. As a result, many individuals have been advised or even prevented from having sex before important fixtures. Research in this area is generally of low quality and mostly involves male participants. There seems to be little evidence to support the theory that sex negatively impacts performance. One study showed that there is no negative effect if the sex occurs at least ten hours before the exercise test, but there is a negative effect if it's less than two hours. It seems reasonable to presume that a late night with hours of sex might not put you in the best physical shape for an endurance event the following morning, due to expended energy and little sleep. However, a 2017 survey of over 4000 Brits by online adult toy business Lovehoney revealed that the average time for sex in the UK is 19 minutes (ten minutes of foreplay and nine minutes of intercourse), which would burn around 70 calories and not put too much of a dent in your energy or sleep.

If pre-race anxiety levels are high, sex can be relaxing and aid sleep, so potentially this could improve performance. There's some evidence that the female orgasm lowers pain thresholds, which if that effect lasted long enough (and we don't know if it does), could be handy when you're hurting in the toughest parts of a race the next day. They say never try anything new on race day and you could add the night before race day too. It's not the best time for new sex positions if you want to avoid a muscular injury. All in all, it's an individual thing – do what works for you and have fun with the trial and error testing!

Q Can running increase your sex drive?

A There are many causes of a low sex drive or libido. While running can't help reduce some of them, such as pain on intercourse, neurological diseases and side-effects of medications, it can help counteract many others. A low libido is often linked to mental health problems, such as anxiety and depression, and we know that regular exercise can help alleviate and treat these (see page 16). Running is a useful tool for managing daily life stress and fatigue, both of which can have a significant effect on how keen you are to have sex. Low self-esteem and poor body image can lower libido, and running has an amazing ability to help people build confidence through goal setting and improving their relationships with their bodies. Regular running is a healthy lifestyle choice and reduces the risk of developing medical conditions that can affect libido, including high blood pressure, obesity and type 2 diabetes.

Did you know?

Erectile dysfunction – problems getting and maintaining erections – affects 40 per cent of men aged 40. By age 70, the figure rises to 70 per cent. If it's happening to you, visit your GP or a sexual health clinic to check for underlying causes.

Q Will running improve sexual performance?

A Studies on this subject rely on surveys and self-reporting so there is always the risk that people don't give accurate answers to questions about their sex lives and exercise habits. One of the larger, more recent studies carried out by the University of California in 2019 surveyed around 3900 men and 2200 women, with an average age of over 40, to determine whether more cardiovascular activity (running, cycling and swimming) each week reduced the likelihood of sexual problems. They found that men doing more cardio exercise each week reported less erectile dysfunction and women exercising more vigorously suffered less sexual dysfunction too, with easier arousal and better orgasm satisfaction. In summary, the more exercise, the greater the sexual performance and satisfaction. The reasons for this are unclear and many factors, both psychological and physical, will have a role, but improved circulation may play a part. Erections rely on an increased blood flow to the penis and women's genitals become engorged with blood during arousal. Remember too that conditions such as high blood pressure, obesity and type 2 diabetes are all causes of erectile dysfunction, which regular running can help to counteract. So, for a great sex life, you are well justified in spending plenty of time in your trainers!

Did you know?

People experience exercise-induced orgasms. Whilst there is little medical evidence to support the claims and poor understanding of why they happen, they seem to be more common in women and more likely during workouts that involve the deep abdominal and pelvic muscles, hence the descriptive term 'coregasm'.

Q Will running affect my fertility and sperm count?

A Sperm-related problems are the most common cause of infertility in men. The sperm may be low in number, abnormal in shape or unable to swim effectively to reach the egg. In the majority of cases the reason for this is unexplained. Lifestyle can affect sperm quality and quantity. Excessive alcohol intake can reduce sperm quality. In overweight or obese people, losing weight can improve sperm counts. We know too that stress and poor sleep can affect sperm production, so using running to maintain good mental health could lead to an improvement. There's strong evidence that smoking reduces sperm counts, so if running helps you to stop smoking then it's having an indirect but significant effect on your fertility. Underlying medical causes for sperm abnormalities include testicular problems such as injury, infection and undescended testicles. Reduced sperm production can result from low testosterone levels due to testicular or pituitary gland tumours. Taking illegal drugs can also affect sperm quality.

What about the direct effect of running on sperm production and quality? A 2017 study from Iran, widely shared in the media, concluded that exercising three times per week can improve sperm quality and number, and that moderate intensity exercise showed the most benefit. There were no changes in sperm in the control group that didn't exercise. This sounds encouraging, but it's wise to consider the limitations of this study. People in all the exercise groups lost weight, so we don't know whether the sperm improvements were due to weight loss or exercise. It's also worth noting that the people in the study didn't exercise prior to taking part, so we can't automatically assume that current runners could improve their sperm counts by running more.

There have been studies showing that excessive exercise can reduce sperm counts. This is particularly frequent in long distance cycling, possibly due to reduced blood flow from saddle pressure and over-heating of the scrotum which may be relevant to endurance runners too. The jury is still very much out on how much of what type of exercise will have the most benefit on sperm production or whether this will actually lead to successful pregnancies. For now, it seems reasonable to say that including moderate amounts of regular running as part of a healthy lifestyle may improve – and won't decrease – your fertility.

According to World Health Organisation guidelines, a normal semen sample will be at least 1.5 millilitres and contain at least 15 million sperm per millilitre with a total of 39 million per ejaculate.

Q My balls ache when I run. Why? And is it harmful?

A There are several reasons why you might get pain in your testicles when you run. The most common is that they simply object to being bounced around. If you're wearing loose fitting boxers or sports shorts, then simply switching to something more supportive could be the answer. You could try tighter underpants or Lycra shorts (on their own or under looser ones, depending on your preference). Compression wear (super-tight clothing that aims to increase blood flow) might be the answer, but if you get any pain or numbness then it means it's too tight. If support doesn't solve the problem or you get pain at other times too, then make an appointment to see your GP to rule out any underlying problem such as inflammation or infection.

Have you heard of a varicocele? There's a little network of veins next to the testicle and if blood flow backs up in these, similar to a varicose vein, then you can develop a squishy swelling called a varicocele, usually on the left testicle due to a slightly increased blood volume compared to the right testicle. They're generally harmless, but because of the increased blood flow during running and the effects of gravity, they can ache and throb during exercise. Supportive underwear can help, but don't self-diagnose. Any lumps or bumps in the scrotum should be checked by a doctor.

Finally, it's possible the pain might be coming from elsewhere and is radiating to your testicles. Pain from the lower back, hernias, urinary tract or thighs can all be felt in the testicles. If in doubt, get checked out and remember that sudden and severe one-sided testicular pain could be torsion, where the testicle has twisted and blood flow is blocked. This is an emergency requiring urgent assessment.

How to check your balls

TRY THIS AT HOME

Examining your testicles once a month will help you to get familiar with how they feel and ensure that you pick up any potentially harmful changes early. Remember that most lumps won't be cancer and if testicular cancer is found early it is nearly always treatable.

Checking yourself is simple. Here's how to do it:

1. Have a warm bath or shower so your scrotal skin is relaxed – checking while you're in the shower is a good idea.
2. Remember, it's normal for one testicle to be larger or hang lower than the other.
3. Standing up, cup your balls in one hand. You can use the other hand to press your penis and the top of your scrotum against your body to keep everything still.
4. Check one testicle at a time and roll the testicle between your thumb and index and middle fingers.
5. The surface should be smooth and uniform. Check for lumps or bumps of any size on the surface of the testicle.
6. At the top and back of each testicle, you will feel a soft, stringy, lumpy area called the epididymis and a firmer, longer, thinner spermatic cord. These are a normal part of the anatomy.
7. If you notice any lumps, changes in size or consistency of the testicle, or any painful areas, then see your doctor.

Q My menstrual cycle really seems to affect my running performance. Is this possible?

A There is an under-representation of women when it comes to sports medicine research so questions like this are difficult to answer. A review in the *British Journal of Sports Medicine* in 2017 found that over 6 million people were included in exercise research studies between 2011 and 2013 and women made up only 39 per cent of that total. Most studies looking at the effect of the menstrual cycle on performance have been carried out with elite athletes as the participants. Measurements such as their oxygen consumption, heart rate and lactic acid production have been monitored, and there's little convincing evidence that performance alters at different times of the cycle. However, if we look at different measures, such as energy levels and motivation, you'll be hard pushed to find a menstruating woman who doesn't report that at certain times of the month running is harder than at others. A study of over 1000 women running the London Marathon in 2015 found that nearly one third of them felt that their menstrual cycle affected their performance and training. With the increasing number of women running and the topic of periods thankfully becoming less taboo, there's more research going on in this area and in non-elite athletes too. Hopefully we'll soon have a much clearer picture of the possible effects and how to counteract them.

Generally, most women report they can run well from the second or third day of their period through until mid-cycle. This seems to be a good time to do high intensity interval and sprint work. Around mid-cycle there is an increased risk of injury, particularly the cruciate ligaments in the knee, probably due to hormonal softening of ligaments. The second half of the cycle seems to be better for endurance runs, but towards the end of this, when pre-menstrual symptoms kick in, motivation and speed take a downturn and body temperature rises. This is a good time for easier runs and cross training. It is a very individual thing and finding what works for you takes time.

Tracking your menstrual cycle

TRY THIS AT HOME

If you're interested in seeing how your menstrual cycle affects your running and training, then start keeping a record of your activity. You can use a simple written diary of your runs. Note down how you felt and any problems you encountered. You could also rate your energy levels, average heart rate and pace. Tally this with your periods and see if there is any pattern throughout the month. There are several menstrual cycle tracking apps available which offer advice on what changes you can make to work with your cycle.

Q My period is due on marathon day! Is there a way I can stop it coming?

A How frustrating! It is possible to delay menstruation using hormonal medications. If you already use the combined oral contraceptive pill and the marathon is falling during your usual pill-free break, then it's easy. Miss the break and carry straight onto the next packet. Be aware that if you use a pill which has seven inactive pills instead of a pill-free break, then you will need to miss out the dummy pills and go straight onto the active pills in a new packet. If you take a pill that has different hormone content on different days (known as a phasic pill) then you should get advice from your practice nurse or a family planning clinic to make sure your contraceptive cover is maintained.

If you aren't on the pill and simply want to delay this period as a one-off, then there is only one drug licensed for this purpose in the UK. It's a progesterone called norethisterone. This is available from your GP and some pharmacies offer it too. You will be asked questions to check it is suitable for you and the possible risks of deep vein thrombosis should be assessed and discussed. Norethisterone needs to be started three days before you expect your period to begin and taken three times a day until after your marathon. You can expect a bleed within three days of stopping it. However, it might not help you perform at your best as it can cause bloating, sluggishness and tender breasts in some women. You could look at using the combined oral contraceptive to control and delay this period, but ideally you would need to start it at least a month or two before the marathon, because irregular bleeding is common in the first few months.

Remember that no method is guaranteed to stop your period and there's no evidence that athletic performance is affected during menstruation, so unless your bleeding is heavy and unmanageable then you may prefer to pad up and run. If heavy periods are frequently affecting your running and racing plans, and you aren't planning to get pregnant, then have a chat with your practice nurse about contraceptive options that might reduce or eliminate your heavy periods.

Q My periods are really heavy, but I don't want to take hormonal contraception. What can I do to stop them affecting my running?

A Many runners have heavy periods. A survey of over 1000 women at the London Marathon in 2015 found that 35.5 per cent of them met the criteria for heavy menstrual bleeding (HMB) and less than half of them had sought medical help for the issue. Interestingly, elite marathon runners were included in this study and 36.7 per cent of them had HMB and just over half said their cycle has an impact on their training and performance. While this doesn't mean you shouldn't run during a period, HMB can make women fear blood leaking onto their clothes and it could potentially cause light-headedness and a lack of energy. It can be associated with cramping pain too. There's also an increased risk of an iron deficiency anaemia with HMB. This may be transient or longer lasting, but can certainly reduce performance (see page 41).

Hormonal contraception can help to control HMB, but not every woman wants to or can use it. If you're concerned about leaking blood, then have a look at some of the 'period underwear' available. These are knickers with the ability to absorb and retain blood. For lighter flows they can be used alone, but with heavy bleeding they can just give you some emergency absorption and therefore reassurance. Running skorts, skirts and dresses can hide bulky sanitary pads if that is a concern. Have a look at menstrual cups. As well as being environmentally friendly, these cups, which fit snuggly into the vagina, can hold up to two or three times as much blood as a tampon. They can be emptied and re-fitted while you're on the go, although you will need to find a loo.

If you think you may be anaemic or heavy bleeding is affecting your daily life and hobbies, then do see your GP. You may need a blood test and potential treatment for anaemia, but options such as using anti-inflammatories or a medication called tranexamic acid to reduce blood flow can be discussed.

Real-life runners

Heavy periods left me exhausted and defeated, both physically and emotionally, and resulted in anaemia. But once my bleeding was resolved, my energy returned and I found the joy in running once again!

Deborah Halliday Mills, writer, runner and mum of boys

Q Can running make my periods stop?

A Sometimes running can lead to amenorrhoea, which is the medical term for absent menstrual periods. Amenorrhoea can be primary (periods never began) or secondary (periods started and then stopped). The definition can vary, but if you have missed periods for between three and six months and you had previously had regular periods, then you would be considered to have secondary amenorrhoea.

There are many causes of secondary amenorrhoea, including pregnancy, menopause, polycystic ovary syndrome, hypothyroidism (underactive thyroid) and stress. It can also be caused by excessive weight loss and excessive exercise, and this is where running may be relevant. If your weight is stable and you are consuming adequate calories to fuel your exercise, then your periods should not be affected, but reduce your calorie intake or increase your activity (or both at once) and you may push the body into a negative energy balance and lose your period. It can be a difficult balance to strike. Without adequate energy the body shuts down some important functions. Menstruation can be one of these. The effects can be widespread in the body and include losing bone strength and being at risk of osteoporosis (see page 146). The point at which this happens is different for every woman. A regular menstrual cycle should be considered as a sign of good health.

If you have amenorrhoea or your periods have become very infrequent (oligomenorrhoea), then although that may feel like a bonus for a runner – no one wants the inconvenience of bleeding – it is important that the cause is addressed, so please see your doctor to discuss it.

Did you know?

A survey published in the *British Medical Journal* in 2001 found that British girls today start their periods (menarche) at an average age of around 13. It's widely believed that the age of menarche has fallen significantly over the years, but this study concluded that compared to girls 20 to 30 years ago, it has only fallen slightly and almost certainly by less than six months.

Q Running gives me spotting. Is this normal?

A Vaginal bleeding between periods is called intermenstrual bleeding (IMB). If the bleeding is just a few drops of blood then it's called spotting. Strenuous exercise can occasionally trigger it. It's unclear exactly why it happens but may be due to fluctuating hormone levels from the exertion. However, it's really important that you don't assume that this is the cause. There are lots of reasons, some of which may be serious, why spotting can happen. IMB can be due to hormonal contraceptives (particularly methods using progesterone), certain medications, pregnancy and infection. Cervical ectropion (delicate areas of cervical tissue), polyps, fibroids and, more rarely, cancer can cause it too. If you have recurrent bleeding between periods then you should make an appointment with your nurse or GP for an assessment. The nurse or doctor will examine your vagina and cervix with a speculum to work out where the bleeding is coming from. They may take some swabs to rule out infection and take a cervical smear test (if it's due). If they have any concerns about the appearance of your cervix or are unsure about the cause of bleeding, then they will refer you to a gynaecologist. Once you have been given the all clear then you can return to running knowing that the bleeding is nothing to worry about.

Q Can I run straight after a cervical smear test?

A There's no reason why you can't go to your cervical screening in your running kit and run straight home afterwards. Sometimes having a smear can make you bleed a little, but this is usually only some light spotting that a panty liner can cope with, so pop one into your knickers before you leave home. Some women have a very sensitive cervix and find smear tests uncomfortable. Any discomfort is, however, usually very short-lived. If you do have any period-type aches afterwards it shouldn't be severe enough to stop you running. The only other thing to bear in mind is that very occasionally having a smear test can make you feel light-headed and dizzy. The cervix can sometimes be very sensitive to contact from the speculum or the swab used to take the sample of cells. This sensitivity can trigger a drop in blood pressure. Again, this is usually short-lived, but you may need a little time to lie or sit and recover slowly. If this happens, particularly if you faint, then you would be better to postpone the run until later in the day when you've had something to eat and drink and are back to your normal self.

Q Should I stop running while I try to get pregnant?

A No. This is a perfect time for you to optimise your health. Regular exercise is a vital component of a healthy lifestyle. It will help you to maintain your weight and we know that many of the risks of pregnancy, such as gestational diabetes (diabetes of pregnancy) and pre-eclampsia (potentially dangerous high blood pressure in pregnancy), are related to being overweight or obese. Being obese can make it harder to get pregnant too. There's no evidence that the high impact nature of running will reduce your risk of conceiving or increase your risk of miscarriage. You need to be having regular periods to conceive and sometimes women who are over-training and/or under-fuelling may have amenorrhoea (an absence of periods). You should be assessed by a specialist if this is the case for you. You will probably be advised to stop or reduce your running for your periods to return.

Getting pregnant can take time, especially as you get older – 18 per cent of couples age 35 to 39 having regular sex haven't conceived after a year of trying. This can be upsetting and the stress-relieving benefits of running can be very useful. Don't forget to maximise your nutrition and take a daily supplement of folic acid while you are trying to get pregnant and until you are 12 weeks pregnant. This will help the early development of your baby's spinal cord and nervous system.

Q How soon can I run after a miscarriage?

A miscarriage can be an emotional experience and spending time running, solo or with friends, can be very helpful as a coping mechanism. You can generally go for a run as soon as you feel able to, but there are a few things to bear in mind. It's normal to bleed after a miscarriage and this can continue for up to three to four weeks. Blood loss should gradually get lighter over this time, but sometimes running can make it a little heavier or seem to make it restart when it had previously stopped. Take things slowly and see how you feel. If your bleeding has been heavy or prolonged, then there is a risk that you may be anaemic. This means you have low levels of red blood cells (see page 41) and as well as feeling very tired you may feel weak, dizzy and breathless on exertion. In this situation it's definitely best to take a few weeks to recover and then restart running very gradually. Very occasionally you can develop an infection after a miscarriage. If you notice your blood loss or discharge is smelly or discoloured, you have increasing abdominal pain or tenderness, or feel sick or shivery, then you may have an infection. Running is not a good idea if you have any of these symptoms and it's important to see your doctor.

Q Is running in pregnancy safe? I don't want to stop.

A If you have an uncomplicated pregnancy, then there is no need for you to stop running unless you want to. There are a few situations where running is dangerous, such as placenta praevia (where the placenta sits right over the cervical opening), early rupture of membranes and recurrent bleeding in the second or third trimester. In these and other complicated pregnancies, and if you have any doubts or concerns about the safety of running for you, then specialist advice is needed. Thankfully, for the majority of women running is safe and beneficial to both mother and baby. Regular exercise – and that includes running – can help to improve and maintain your physical fitness, which is important for labour. It can also help to reduce the risk of pre-eclampsia, lower the risk of gestational diabetes, and help you to feel mentally and physically well during your pregnancy.

Breasts grow and can become tender, so you will probably need a new sports bra at least once during your pregnancy. You might find your feet grow too! It's important to keep well hydrated, adequately fuelled and to listen to your body. If you keep your exercise to a moderate intensity, where you can talk while you're running, and to sessions of up to 45 minutes, then you don't need to worry about over-exerting yourself. Warm up well, take breaks and stop when you need to. Stop running and get advice from your midwife or doctor if you experience any of the following symptoms:

- Abdominal pain.
- Vaginal bleeding.
- Fluid leaking from your vagina.
- Painful, regular contractions
- Chest pain.
- Dizziness.
- Headache.
- Calf pain or swelling.

A few women run right up to their delivery date, but others find that running becomes difficult and prefer other lower-impact activities such as swimming in the later months. You might find that your growing bump becomes uncomfortable, that running makes indigestion worse or that you lose your sense of balance. Whatever your reason to stop running (and it can be frustrating if you are keen to carry on), you should know that any exercise you do is beneficial and running will always be there when you are ready to try again.

Did you know?

The Chief Medical Officers' Guidelines 2019 for physical activity during pregnancy are basically the same as those for non-pregnant women. They still recommend 150 minutes of moderate intensity activity every week and muscle-strengthening activities twice per week. They advise that if you're already active you can keep going and if you're inactive then you should start gradually. Listening to your body, adapting your exercise and taking care not to bump your bump are the other key pieces of advice.

Q How soon after giving birth can I run?

A The traditional answer to this is after your six-week check with your GP. In reality, this is very unhelpful. It is much more complicated than this and for the majority of women this is far too soon. The desire to be back out running can be intense, but equally it can be the last thing on your mind. Every woman is different and no one should feel under any pressure to get back to running until they want to.

Returning to running too soon or too rapidly can cause future problems of incontinence and pelvic organ prolapse. This is true for both vaginal and Caesarean section deliveries. Even if you don't feel you have any pelvic floor weakness (see page 98), you will benefit from returning to exercise in the correct way.

The Returning to Running Postnatal Guidelines, written by three physiotherapists with huge experience and knowledge in this field, were published in March 2019. Their expert opinion is that it's not advisable to run before 12 weeks postnatal or beyond this if there are symptoms or signs of pelvic floor dysfunction. They recommend allowing your body the time it needs to heal, and following a low-impact exercise programme to restore your pelvic floor and abdominal muscles to full strength before beginning high-impact exercise. Ideally this would be a guided, personalised plan supervised by a women's health physiotherapist. Exercises can begin immediately after your baby has been born, with gentle walking, core and pelvic floor muscle work. They suggest building up to power walking, resistance work and some weights work at six to eight weeks, and further progression to swimming and spinning from weeks eight to 12. Assuming both core and pelvic floor muscle strength have been adequately restored, running can commence gradually, from 12 weeks. A Couch to 5k programme is an ideal way to do this, because it combines short periods of running with walking. Any woman who experiences urinary or faecal incontinence, a heaviness or pressure in the pelvic area or a bulging of their abdomen, suggesting that the abdominal muscles are separated, should seek a referral to a women's health physiotherapist for assessment and rehabilitation.

Patience is key. Running is an ideal way to guard against and treat postnatal depression, and will help you to regain your fitness and sense of self when the demands a baby places on you are intense. However, a planned and gradual return to running is the best way to ensure your body will be fit and able to run problem-free for years to come.

Q I'm ready to get back to running, but I'm still breastfeeding my baby. Is this OK?

A study back in 1991 showed a significantly increased amount of lactic acid in breast milk ten minutes after maximal intensity exercise, but, by 30 minutes, the levels were almost the same as those pre-exercise. Most women will not be exercising at their maximum capacity and other studies have shown no increase in lactic acid in breast milk after moderate intensity exercise. There is no evidence to suggest that lactic acid in breast milk is harmful to babies anyway and maternal exercise hasn't been shown to have any negative effect on the growth of breast-fed babies. A study looking at whether babies refuse breast milk due to potentially altered taste from lactic acid did not show any difference in the baby's acceptance of the milk one hour after moderate or high intensity exercise. To date, the evidence is reassuring that running and breast feeding are entirely compatible. The benefits of a happy, exercising mother mustn't be underestimated. Here are my top tips for running and breast feeding:

1 Feed your baby or express some milk before you run. Your breasts will be lighter. You can then relax knowing your baby has just eaten and you might even have time for a shower when you get back before the next feed!

2 Wear your most supportive sports bra with breast pads if you're prone to leaking. If your nipples are sore, then protect them with some lanolin or petroleum jelly.

3 Drink plenty of fluid before and after your run. Running is
   thirsty work and so is breast feeding.
4 Make sure your diet is top notch with lots of fresh and iron-rich
   foods, and take 10 micrograms of vitamin D daily.
5 Be aware that some of the hormones still circulating in your
   bloodstream post-partum may relax your joints and ligaments,
   and potentially put you at increased risk of injury.
6 If you use sports supplements to fuel longer runs, then watch
   out for those containing large amounts of caffeine in case
   they affect your baby's sleep. Up to 200 milligrams of caffeine
   daily is the recommended amount while breastfeeding,
   which is equivalent to two cups of instant coffee or one cup of
   Americano.

Did you know?

The average age of the menopause in the UK is 51 but the symptoms of the
peri-menopause, which is the time leading up to the menopause, usually
start when a woman is in her 40s.

Q Will running help me with my peri-menopausal symptoms?

A You reach the menopause when your periods have stopped
for 12 months. The time leading up to this is called the
perimenopause. The heavy or irregular bleeding coupled with
tender breasts and fatigue often experienced by women during this
time, which lasts for an average of four years, don't exactly inspire you
to put on your trainers, but it's definitely worth it if you can. Running
during the perimenopause can help to counteract some of the many
symptoms you might experience. For example, bloating, headaches

and joint pain can all be reduced by exercise and, although you might think running would make you more tired, it can actually give you an energy boost.

A Cochrane review (a systematic review of primary health research) in 2014 found insufficient evidence to show whether exercise would help with hot flushes and night sweats. A small study in 2016 found that women who trained to increase their fitness experienced fewer sweats and flushes, but more research needs to be done to confirm exactly what type and how much exercise is needed for this purpose.

Running will help to maintain and build bone and muscle mass, both of which decline rapidly from this point on. Strong bones and muscles will improve your future health and increasing your muscle mass will help to counteract the natural weight gain that can happen around the menopause too, so it's a good idea to add in some work with weights alongside your running.

Low mood, irritability and mood swings are a common peri-menopausal symptom, and this is where running really comes into its own, offering a natural way to boost mood, release tension and deliver a sense of wellbeing (see page 5). It can improve concentration, focus and sleep too, so running is a really useful tool for managing the mental health effects of the menopause.

Real-life runners

I started running in my early 50s after discovering the positive impact exercise had on my perimenopause. It has really helped my increased anxiety, sleep problems and self-confidence. Running has brought me joy, friendship and a sense of purpose.

Jo, mum of two grown up sons, lives on the edge of the Yorkshire Dales

TOP TIPS FOR A HEALTHY RUNNER'S REPRODUCTIVE SYSTEM

- Attend screenings such as cervical and antenatal screenings.
- Perform regular self-examination, for example on breasts and testicles.
- Visit a sexual health clinic for a screen for sexually transmitted diseases if you have any symptoms you're worried about or for reassurance if you have ever had unprotected sex.
- Practise safe sex.
- Report any unusual bleeding, lumps or other changes to your GP.
- Lead a healthy lifestyle. Don't smoke, maintain a healthy weight and eat a healthy diet full of fresh fruit and vegetables. Keep exercising regularly.
- Take your time returning to running after childbirth. Follow a core and pelvic floor rehabilitation programme and then build up slowly from walking.
- Consider tracking your menstrual cycle if you want to identify any effects on your training.

FURTHER HELP AND ADVICE

Menopause Matters: www.menopausematters.co.uk
The Miscarriage Association: www.miscarriageassociation.org.uk
Male cancer – Orchid: www.orchid-cancer.org.uk
Relate: www.relate.org.uk
Sexual Advice Association: www.sexualadviceassociation.co.uk
Cervical cancer – Jo's Trust: www.jostrust.org.uk
Gynaecological cancers – Eve Appeal: www.eveappeal.org.uk

CHAPTER 7

······································

THE MUSCULOSKELETAL SYSTEM

The musculoskeletal system is made up of bones, joints, muscles, tendons, ligaments and more, all of which give our body structure and shape. The system from our toes to our finger tips is truly an incredible feat of engineering. It allows us to perform large movements, such as running and jumping and tiny, intricate movements, such as threading a needle. Force, tension and pressure are applied in multiple directions at once, but our body structure is light enough for us to move around freely. What's even more amazing is that the body has its own systems to repair and strengthen any weaknesses so it can perform even better the next time. So is the act of running good or bad for the musculoskeletal system and what can we do to keep it in optimum condition?

Public Health England report that every year 20 per cent of people see their GP about a musculoskeletal problem and over 17 million people in the UK are affected by musculoskeletal conditions. Of course, doing exercise puts you at risk of injury and might lead to you having to use the health service, but the evidence is overwhelming that keeping physically active is good for your health. Not only will you live longer, but you'll lower your risk of disability from osteoarthritis, falls and hip fractures, and increase the likelihood that you can remain living independently and pain free.

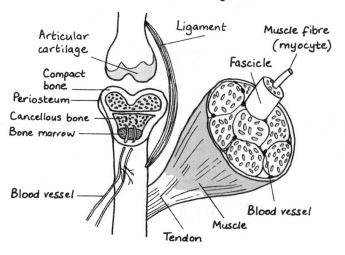

The Musculoskeletal System

All the elements of the musculoskeletal system are living. Our bones, far from being the inert, hollow structure you may visualise, are in fact alive. Bones are constantly being broken down (to release minerals such as calcium) and reformed to keep them strong. They're also filled with bone marrow, which makes new blood cells. Nerves and blood vessels run through and over bones to nourish them, so they're far from static. Muscles are made up of cells called myocytes that are arranged into long strands of muscle fibres. Myocytes are packed with mitochondria, which are the power packs supplying energy to the cells. With incredible endurance and strength potential we need to take care of our muscles and do what we can to preserve their integrity and mass, especially as we age. Tendons are what anchor muscles to bones. They're formed from the tough outer coating of muscles. When the muscle contracts, the tendon pulls on the bone and the bone moves. Ligaments are tough fibrous bands which attach bones to bones and their role is to stabilise joints. For example, in the knee there are ligaments to stop the knee slipping sideways, forwards and backwards. If a joint dislocates then the ligament hasn't done its job and has overstretched or torn, allowing the bones to slip out of place.

Running certainly stresses the musculoskeletal system, but stress isn't necessarily a bad thing, because it's only by stressing something that it's made stronger. However, stresses in the wrong direction and inadequate time for recovery can lead to a breakdown of the system. As runners we need to respect our musculoskeletal system and do what we can to ensure we're giving it all it needs to function at its best. Let's start with muscles, move on to bones and joints, and then look more specifically at knees, feet, ankles, hips and the spine. There is quite a bit of crossover in all these sections so read the whole chapter rather than just one section.

MUSCLES

Q Why do my muscles hurt so much the day after a long run, and how can I ease the pain and stiffness?

A You may have heard the term DOMS. This stands for Delayed Onset Muscle Soreness and the typical picture is of a runner standing at the top of a set of stairs the day after a marathon and wondering how on earth they're going to get down them!
Any time you push your muscles to their limits, whether through endurance or strength workouts, you'll probably feel some DOMS. We used to think that the pain was due to a build-up of lactic acid in muscles, but we now know that this usually clears within a couple of hours of stopping exercise. Instead, we think DOMS is due to micro-tears in muscle fibres – tiny rips that happen during intense exercise. As the body heals the tears, muscles become a little inflamed and swollen, making them stiff, sore and tender. It's important to prioritise recovery, to allow muscles to repair and strengthen themselves for your next run.

What can help the pain of DOMS? Time is the biggest factor. It's usually gone within three to five days. There's no evidence that warming up or stretching will reduce DOMS happening, but being well trained to run the selected distance certainly will, so following a gradually increasing training plan is the best preventative. Ice baths straight after exercise might be beneficial and so might a post-race massage, but the evidence is mixed. If you have DOMS, try light exercise, warm baths, ice packs, gentle massage, compression wear and paracetamol to get you through the worst days and return slowly to running when you're ready.

Q I'm running my first marathon and don't want to be one of those runners you see at the side of the course with bad muscle cramp. Why does it happen and how can I prevent it?

Muscle fibres contract (shorten) and relax (lengthen) in turn when a muscle is used. Sometimes the muscle gets stuck in a contracted state and that's when you get the excruciating pain of cramp. It's a pain that's impossible to ignore, as demonstrated by runners having to stop when they'd otherwise just tough it out. There are multiple causes of cramps, including dehydration, low mineral levels (sodium, potassium, calcium and magnesium) and poor circulation. Cramps can sometimes be due to underlying medical conditions such as diabetes, thyroid disorders and medications, and they're also more common in pregnancy.

But what causes a cramp in an otherwise well runner who has kept hydrated, replaced their electrolytes and doesn't have any medical conditions? The answer seems to lie in the theory of altered neuromuscular control and there is a growing acceptance of this explanation for exercise-associated muscle cramps (EAMC). Muscles contain stretch receptors called muscle spindles which detect muscle length, relay that information to the brain and spinal cord, and activate muscle contraction. At the same time, structures called the Golgi tendon organs detect tension in muscles and tendons (which attach muscle to bone), and prevent too much loading by inhibiting muscle activation. When there is an imbalance in these messages and the muscle spindle messages overwhelm the Golgi tendon organ ones, then involuntary muscle contractions occur. This imbalance can happen in fatigued muscles, is probably exacerbated by heat and is more likely in undertrained runners.

If you get cramp the best thing to do is to stop and passively stretch the affected muscle. Passive stretching means the muscle itself is not doing the work. The easiest way to passively stretch your hamstring is to lie down, and get someone else to lift your leg off the ground and raise it towards your head. You can passively stretch your own calf by taking hold of your foot and flexing it. Drink fluids to negate any dehydration and let your body temperature slowly return to normal. Most importantly, prevent cramp by training sensibly and gradually for your marathon, practising your fuelling and adjusting your expectations according to the weather conditions on the day.

Did you know?

Leg cramps in the evening and at night can be part of Restless Leg Syndrome, a frustrating condition when the sufferer has the overriding desire to move their legs around. Aching, itching, jerking and tingling can all be present. The cause is unclear, although sometimes there's an underlying medical condition such as an underactive thyroid, iron deficiency or diabetes. Runners can experience restless legs after a particularly long, hard run.

Q Why am I better at running slower over long distances than I am at sprinting short ones?

A Muscles contain two different types of muscle fibres: slow-twitch fibres and fast-twitch fibres. The slow-twitch fibres, also known as type 1 or red fibres, contract slowly, don't fatigue easily and are used in endurance exercise. Fast-twitch fibres, also called type 2 or white fibres, contract quickly, tire rapidly and are designed for explosive movements like jumping and sprinting. We're born with a certain amount of each, usually around half and half, but the ratio of each is largely what determines our strongest events when it comes to running. If your muscles are packed with fast-twitch fibres (think Usain Bolt) then sprinting is probably your niche. If, however, you have a higher percentage of slow-twitch muscle fibres (think Paula Radcliffe), then you may be more suited to marathon distance. Genetics have a large role to play in this, but you can't ignore the environmental factors and your ability to target training at the different fibres. The evidence is mixed as to whether you can convert one fibre into another, but you can certainly work and train with what you have.

As we age, we naturally lose muscle mass and this seems to be predominantly a reduction in size of the type 2, fast-twitch fibres. This explains why we get slower with age and highlights the need to include strength training, particularly in later life, to negate this loss. Interestingly, a study in Finland in 2000 found that an aptitude for endurance events (with a higher percentage of slow-twitch fibres) and continuing that activity through life gave some protection against coronary heart disease that was not seen in those who had an aptitude for power speed events. It seems our muscle fibres may influence more than which events we sign up for.

Q I'm confused about stretching! Should I do it before running, after running or not even bother?

A It's easy to get confused when the advice we're given keeps changing! This topic is quite controversial, but we seem to have settled into an acceptance that traditional static stretching isn't beneficial before a run, but might be afterwards. Stretching cold muscles before you run won't increase your performance or reduce your risk of injury. Warming up rather than stretching should be your priority before a run (see page 226). Brisk walking and slow running is enough and you can add what we call dynamic stretches to prepare your muscles and joints for running. A dynamic stretch is a stretch that's done in a controlled way while a muscle is in motion and takes a joint through its full range of movement. Dynamic stretches for runners include arm swings, hip swings and lunges. Traditional static stretches can be done after your run when muscles are warm and pliable, to lengthen muscles, particularly if you have a known tightness. Stretching out your calves, quads and hamstrings can improve flexibility. Again, there's still some uncertainty as to how crucial this is in terms of recovery or injury prevention, but it does at least provide some social time at the end of a group run!

Q Do runners really need to do strength and conditioning?

A I think the majority of runners feel a bit guilty, because they know they probably should do some muscle strength and conditioning work, but prefer to just go for a run instead. It's easy to think it's unnecessary and that running is enough, but there are many benefits to doing strength and conditioning. Having strong muscles helps you to run with good technique – more efficiently with increased power and less risk of injury. No runner is going to turn those benefits down.

A strong core will hold you upright, allowing you to fully expand your lungs, keep your pelvis and hips stable for ideal running technique, and fire up the often lazy and weak gluteus maximus muscles. Strong arm muscles will help power your sprint finish and drive you up hills. Strong muscles around a joint such as the knee will help to take the impact off the cartilage and bones in the joint. Having a regular strength and conditioning routine will allow you to focus on individual muscle groups and work them against resistance. That may simply be your own bodyweight, increased resistance from a band or a weight.

Take the glute muscles, for example. If you spend a lot of your day sitting, then it's likely that you have weak glutes. When muscles aren't used, the nerve pathways that stimulate them switch off. When you then run, the glute muscles don't fire and you're missing out on the power of the biggest muscles in the body. Spending some time re-igniting those pathways, learning to use your glutes and strengthening them with the addition of weights will lead to rewards in your running.

It's important to work all the major muscle groups so you have balance on the front and back of your body and limbs. If you work your back then you need to work your abdominals. If you work your glutes then you need to work your quads (quadriceps or front of thigh muscles) etc. You only need to do it once or twice a week and there's no need to join a gym. Runners can have a perfectly good work out at home with little or no equipment. There's evidence that heavy resistance training is more effective than low resistance with lots of repetitions, so don't be afraid to go short and heavy.

We also know that both muscle and bone mass decrease with age, and regular muscle-strengthening work will help to counteract both of these and keep you running fit for the future as well as the present.

Q Foam rolling hurts so much. Can it really be good for me?

A Is it possible that the pain of what genuinely feels like torture from a roll of hard foam will help your running? Should it be an established part of caring for your muscles or is it just a popular trend without good evidence of benefit? In summary, there's no clear answer. Foam rolling may well help to ease sore, tired muscles and increase their flexibility, but there's not sufficient evidence yet to say exactly when and for how long we should foam roll to make a difference to our recovery and performance. So, like many of these techniques, if it seems to help you, then carry on doing it, but don't rely on it to knock time off your PB.

Foam rolling is effectively a type of deep tissue massage. Fascia is the fibrous tissue that encloses and lies between bundles of muscle fibres (you will have seen this slightly shiny sheet of strong tissue if you're used to preparing the Sunday roast). It's thought that with repetitive movements such as running, the fascia can thicken and stick to the underlying muscle, which restricts its movement. When you foam roll you compress your muscle against the roller using your body weight. This is said to free up those sticky areas, make the fascia more pliable, and allow the fascia and muscles to glide freely against each other again. The medical term for this is myofascial release.

In addition, foam rolling may warm up muscles before a workout by causing friction and after a run it may speed up recovery by increasing blood flow. There's also a theory that the benefits aren't just due to myofascial release and may be in part or fully attributable to the effect that rolling has on pain receptors. Information is transmitted to the brain when the nerves are stimulated due to temporarily increased pain. Messages then come back to the nervous system to relax the muscles and that feeling of release is felt. Some therapists argue that foam rolling should not be painful and that if it is then you're doing it wrong. They advise not rolling directly over ligaments, joints and bones and sticking to more gentle rolling over large muscles groups, such as the glutes and hamstrings. This means that rolling up and down directly over that IT band isn't a good idea. There's so much we still don't know about foam rolling and its popularity has spread faster than the evidence for it.

BONES AND JOINTS

Q Will running damage my knees?

A The million-dollar question and the reason many people give for not wanting to run! To answer it in one sentence: a recreational runner of a healthy weight, who trains sensibly, allows adequate recovery, runs with good biomechanics and isn't pre-disposed to osteoarthritis does not need to worry about damaging their knees.

Knees are cleverly designed to absorb impact, keep moving smoothly and to repair any stresses or damage that comes their way. Bones respond well to impact and weight-bearing exercise can increase bone strength. Maintaining a healthy weight (and running can help you achieve that) will mean that the load placed on the knee joint isn't excessive. Training sensibly and building up your running miles gradually will make sure the joint and the muscles around it have time to strengthen and adapt. Ensuring you have rest days and time for recovery will allow for joint repair processes. As you get older, you'll need to prioritise more time for recovery because repair processes slow with age.

If you run with poor technique or an injury which alters your posture and running gait, then you risk potentially damaging your knees due to stresses being put on the knees in a direction which they were not designed for. While the knee can cope with an awful lot, excessive miles with abnormal biomechanics over time may lead to damage.

Whether or not you will develop significant, symptomatic osteoarthritis (OA) in your knees has more to do with your genetics than how much you run. The truth is that we are all different. There's no magic number for how many miles we can run and how much recovery we need, and there's insufficient evidence to say that running will damage your knees. Remember: you are more likely to have problems with your knees if you are inactive than if you are a runner.

An interesting study done in 2019 took 82 middle-aged adults who were running their first marathon and scanned their knees six months before and two weeks after their marathon. During the four-month training programme 11 dropped out, but 71 went on to run their marathons. Six months before the marathon, most of them had some changes to their knee structures linked with the onset of osteoarthritis, even though they didn't have any symptoms. After the marathon there was an improvement in some of these changes in the ends of the tibia and femur, and a worsening of the changes in the cartilage of the patella. Any worsening was still asymptomatic and we don't know in the longer term whether these changes persisted or improved. Potentially, if we could counteract that patella damage in some way, perhaps with injury prevention exercises, then we could say that middle-aged runners who start running a marathon could protect their knees from future osteoarthritis.

Did you know?

There are over 206 bones in the adult body. Children have more, but many bones fuse together as they grow.

Q I'm overweight. Will running harm my joints?

A Running places much more impact onto a joint than walking. Joints are well-designed to carry load and absorb impact, but there does come a point at which excess weight will put strain on a joint and potentially lead to damage. Some exercise will always be better than no exercise and you are more likely to have joint problems if you are inactive. Being overweight doesn't mean you shouldn't run, but you do need to be careful, because it's a high-impact activity and people who are overweight are at higher risk of osteoarthritis. Running can help you reach and maintain a healthy weight, if that's your goal, but not every overweight person runs to lose weight and it's important to acknowledge that. You do, however, need to take care of your joints to prevent damage and injury. You can do this by building up your distances gradually, and allowing rest and recovery time between runs to enable joint and muscle repair. Running with a good technique, and doing strength and conditioning exercises, is important too. Don't ignore twinges. You are asking a lot of your body so become very self-aware, listen to it and take prompt action to avoid long-term problems.

Q I've got some osteoarthritis in my knees. Am I OK to keep running?

A Being told you have osteoarthritis (OA) by your doctor can be very upsetting, particularly if you are a runner, but it may not be as bad as you think. First of all, it's important to know that what is seen on an x-ray may not correlate with what you feel. You can have quite significant pain from your knees and have an almost normal x-ray. Conversely, you can have marked arthritic changes on your x-ray and not experience any pain from your knees at all. How your knees actually feel is more important and doctors won't usually order an x-ray when they suspect OA, because it can be unhelpful.

OA used to be called the 'wear and tear' arthritis, but this implies someone has worn out their joints through being active. Really it should be called the 'wear and repair' arthritis, because your joint is changing and adapting in order to keep it mobile and flexible. The worst thing you can do if you have OA is to avoid using your joint through fear of wearing it out further.

There's good evidence that exercise should be used as a treatment for OA. Resistance exercises are particularly helpful for reducing pain and stiffness, and a training plan containing flexibility and aerobic exercise, as well as strength work, is most likely to improve pain and maintain function in the knee. All exercises need to be done consistently and regularly or the effect will wear off. Physical activity can work as well as, and in some cases better than, pain medications in OA, and is clearly a safer and better long-term option.

Exercise is definitely essential for your future joint health, but how your OA is going to affect your running depends on the severity of your condition and the degree of pain that you have. This is a very individual thing and you will need to discuss it with your doctor. If you have severe OA with little or no meniscus left (the menisci are the shock-absorbing pads in the knee joint) then effectively you have bone on bone contact and running may not be advised. If, however, you have mild disease with few symptoms then running, alongside lots of strength and flexibility work, may be a good way forward for you. Consider including some low-impact cross training such as cycling or swimming into your training plan, running off road when you can to reduce impact and adding in some extra recovery days. Be guided by any pain or swelling and increase or decrease your activities accordingly. Don't immediately despair. With advice, trial and error and determination, a diagnosis of OA doesn't always mean the end of your running career.

Real-life runners

When the surgeon told me I must not try to run again after a knee replacement, I didn't disobey, I just sort of forgot. After three years of cautious build-up, I was winning my age-group again. Now, two and a half years after the other knee was replaced, I'm back to age-graded 80 per cent. It takes care, patience and a touch of stubbornness, but at 80 I'm a runner again. And the latest medical research agrees with me.

Roger Robinson, former England and New Zealand international, author of *When Running Made History* and winner of an award from the American Academy of Orthopaedic Surgeons for his writing about running on knee replacements

Q Will running help prevent osteoporosis?

A Weight-bearing exercises such as running are perfect for strengthening bones, because the jolt on impact with the ground stimulates bone production. Bones are constantly being made by cells called osteoblasts and broken down by osteoclasts, so we need to make sure that the formation exceeds the destruction in order to maintain our bone mass. Exercise is an ideal way to do this and as well as weight-bearing exercise, muscle-strengthening exercises will improve bone health too. When you're using a muscle against resistance such as with a weight or resistance band, the tendon, which attaches the muscle to bone, tugs on the bone, which stimulates bone formation.

Osteoporosis is a condition that affects approximately one in three women and one in 12 men. When bone destruction exceeds bone formation, then bone mass reduces. Reduced bone mass is called osteopenia and, when it falls below a certain level, osteoporosis is diagnosed. The bones are weaker, more fragile and prone to fracture with minimal or no trauma. Common bones to break include the wrist, spine and hips, and all can have significant consequences on an individual's life and future, including the possibility of long-term pain and reduced mobility, so we need to do all we can to prevent osteoporosis.

Q Is it OK to run if I have osteoporosis?

A Running is a great impact activity for maintaining bone mass, but if you have established osteoporosis then you will need to get individual advice from your doctor. Most people will be able to carry on running. Exercise is an important part of your treatment and by exercising more you may actually see an improvement in your bone mass. Occasionally, if you have more advanced disease, particularly in your spine, then your doctor may feel the risks of running outweigh the benefits and you will have to adapt what you do. There's a great factsheet on exercising with osteoporosis available online from the Royal Osteoporosis Society. It explains how important exercise is if you have osteoporosis and gives good advice about exercising safely.

Did you know?

By the age of 18 you will have 90 per cent of your bone mass. It reaches its peak strength around 30 with men reaching a higher bone mass than women. Bone mass then gradually declines as you age, with a sharp drop in women around the time of the menopause. Women tend to lose bone from a younger age and at a faster rate than men.

Q What are shin splints?

A The answer to this isn't as straightforward as you may think, because we don't actually know! Some runners, particularly beginners and those who have rapidly increased their mileage, develop pain and tenderness in the shin area on the front of their lower legs. Shin splints are also called medial tibial stress syndrome.

The tibia is the name of the larger of the two bones in the lower leg and the medial side is the inner part where the pain is most often felt. The condition seems to result from an increase in stress in this area, but there's confusion as to the cause, with some believing it results from tiny amounts of bleeding between the periosteum (the outer layer of bone) and where the muscles attach. Some studies using scans have found no actual changes to the bones or tendons that explain the symptoms of pain and tenderness. It certainly seems to be an over-use injury that starts gradually, is worse when running and is eased by rest.

While we may not fully understand the causes of the pain, there are certain factors that seem to make people more likely to get shin splints, and these can be addressed to help prevent them occurring and enhance recovery. People who are overweight are more at risk due to the increased load on the lower legs. Beginners are particularly vulnerable too, especially if they increase distance rapidly without allowing sufficient time for the lower leg muscles to adapt. If you've had shin splints before then you're more at risk of getting them again and women are affected more than men. These two factors may well be linked to biomechanics and it seems that weaknesses or imbalances in the hip and core muscles may have a role to play. Interestingly, there's also some evidence from a small study in high school athletes that running with a lower cadence (slow step rate) might put you at higher risk of shin splints than running with a higher cadence.

Q I've got shin splints. How long should I rest for?

A Rest is important and you need to wait until you are pain free with no tenderness on pressing your shins, and no pain on walking and jumping, before you begin to run again. You can apply ice to your shins (see page 209) and take pain killers such as paracetamol or ibuprofen if you need to. It will probably take between two to four weeks for the pain to go. During that time it's thought to be OK to exercise if what you're doing isn't causing you pain. Cycling and swimming are ideal things to try.

If you think your shin splints were just due to increasing your distance too rapidly then you can manage your own gradual return to running. However, if you have had shin splints before or you think there may be an underlying cause, such as your running gait, then it would be advisable to seek an assessment from a physiotherapist with expertise in running. They will be able to look at the bigger picture, spot weaknesses that may be triggering your shin pain and devise a recovery programme for you. They may recommend that you are fitted with orthotics for your shoes to correct pronation of your feet as this can be a cause for some people, but it's a little controversial as to how big an issue this is.

Returning to running gradually and slowly increasing the load on your tibia is the key. It's a good idea to start on softer ground, such as grass, and consider doing some of your runs every week off-road in the future. Strengthening your calf muscles may reduce the recurrence of shin splints. Calf raises while holding weights in your hands is a simple exercise you can do at home.

Be guided by pain. Don't try to run through it. If it's flaring up again, then return to your cross training and try again after another period of rest. If it's recurrent, then seek an expert opinion to look for an underlying cause and to rule out a stress fracture.

Healthy bones

It's vital to take steps to maintain your bone mass, particularly if you are a women around menopausal age. Here are some simple things you can do to maximise your bone health:

- Run regularly. Weight-bearing exercise will strengthen bones.
- Add muscle-strengthening to your training plan. This helps to stimulate bone growth too.
- Stop smoking. Smokers have a higher risk of osteoporosis.
- Cut down on alcohol. People who drink a lot of alcohol have a higher risk of osteoporosis. Stick to a maximum of 14 units per week.

continued overleaf ▶

- Eat a healthy diet to give you all the vitamins and minerals needed for bone health. Include calcium rich foods such as dairy products, green leafy vegetables and almonds.
- Consider taking a Vitamin D supplement. We get most of our vitamin D from sunlight and it can be hard to get enough from our diet, so you may want to consider taking a daily 10 microgram supplement, especially in the winter months.

Q How do I know if I've got a stress fracture?

A Repeated over-use and overloading of bone can sometimes lead to stress fractures where bone has literally cracked from overwork. They account for 15 to 20 per cent of musculoskeletal injuries in runners and are most common in feet, shins, knees, hips and the pelvis. Women are affected more than men and if you have had a stress fracture before, or have osteoporosis, then you are at a higher risk of having one.

The pain from a stress fracture tends to come on suddenly, in contrast to the more gradual onset of shin splints pain. It will get worse when you run, whereas many musculoskeletal conditions seem to loosen up and ease once you're running. It also tends to hurt when you aren't running and pain at rest is a red flag that there's something significant going on. Another red flag is that you can identify a point where the bone is tender. Shin splints tend to give a diffuse area of tenderness, but you can literally 'put your finger on it' with a stress fracture. You might also notice some swelling at the site of the tenderness or further down your leg.

Like shin splints, stress fractures tend to occur when people over do it, running long distances frequently, often without adequate recovery time. Whether certain running styles, such as heel striking or forefoot landing, put you at more risk is open for debate and needs more research. Similarly, it's not possible to say whether cushioning in shoes is definitely protective either.

Stress fractures don't always show up on an x-ray so may require more detailed scans, such as CT, MRI or bone scans. If a fracture is confirmed, then rest is essential. It will usually take around eight weeks for it to heal up. Going back to running too soon can cause more damage and lead to a more prolonged time off. Cross training that doesn't trigger pain is allowed, so you can still maintain your fitness, but do check with your doctor what is suitable for you and when. A gradual return to running is essential and it's advisable to see a physiotherapist for a biomechanical assessment, strength exercises and a graded return to exercise.

KNEES

Q What is runner's knee?

A Rather than being a single diagnosis, runner's knee is the term given to a variety of conditions that cause pain in the knees of runners. You may hear it called patellofemoral pain syndrome (PFPS). It tends to affect beginner runners or those who are increasing their distance and frequency of running. The pain is felt in, behind or around the knee cap (patella) and is often worse when running downhill or squatting. Despite the location of the pain, the problem isn't usually from the knee itself. Hip, thigh, calf, foot and even core muscle weaknesses, tightness and imbalances all affect the alignment and function of the knee, and can result in knee pain. For example, if you are sedentary for large parts of your day then you will probably have weak glute muscles, which can result in the knees moving towards a knock-knee position when you run. This is particularly true for women. A weak core and poor stabilisation of your pelvis can lead to your hip dropping when you land, which puts an uneven stress on your knee too.

Treatment initially focuses on letting the acute pain settle and then correcting the underlying problem. You may need a physiotherapist assessment to instruct you. Working on core strength, and hip and leg muscle strength, is vital. Try exercises such as squats, glute bridges and clam shells, (see figure below) either with or without a resistance band.

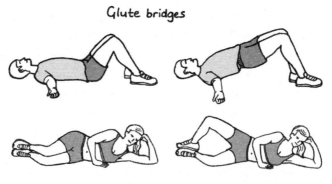

Glute bridges

Clam shells

If the issue is more to do with your foot mechanics, then get fitted for running shoes in a specialist store with a video analysis of your gait. Runner's knee can be overcome, but it may take some determination to solve it. Don't give up, though, and keep doing your strength exercises as part of a weekly schedule to stop it recurring.

FEET AND ANKLES

Q I get pins and needles in my feet when I run long distances and they sometimes go completely numb. Why is that and how can I stop it?

A Pins and needles and foot numbness, either whole or partial, are surprisingly common complaints. Thankfully, the cause isn't usually anything to worry about, but it's a very odd sensation when you're running and can't feel your foot. The first thing to consider is how your shoes are laced. Tight lacing will stop your foot moving in your shoe and help prevent blisters (see page 178), but it can cause problems. Superficial skin nerves easily become compressed, resulting in tingling and numbness, particularly when feet swell on long distances. It may simply be a case of loosening your laces slightly or investigating different lacing techniques.

Lacing Up Trainers

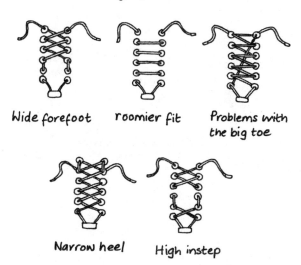

Wide forefoot   roomier fit   Problems with the big toe

Narrow heel   High instep

Try these different lacing techniques if you are struggling with foot numbness, blisters or damaged toenails.

Sometimes going up a size in your trainer or choosing a wider fit will help. A complete change of trainer brand and style might also be the answer. It can take time to find the perfect fit and our feet do change over the years, so it's not necessarily one brand and size for life.

Nerves can also be compressed by the surrounding structures, such as swollen or tight muscles, cysts or bony overgrowths. Often the place where they are compressed is higher up the body than where the numbness is felt. A good example of this is a numbness under the foot which comes from a slipped disc in the lower spine. Sometimes a foot numbness can be due to a thickening of nerve tissue called a Morton's neuroma (see page 158).

Rarely, foot numbness, also called peripheral neuropathy, can be due to an underlying medical condition. Peripheral nerves (those in the extremities of the body) can be damaged and not function properly due to a range of underlying causes, including diabetes (most common cause), an underactive thyroid, excessive alcohol and deficiencies of certain vitamins, particularly vitamin B12. If both feet are numb, then this makes a medical condition more likely. If you've tried to solve your foot numbness yourself with no luck or you have other symptoms alongside it, then you should see your doctor.

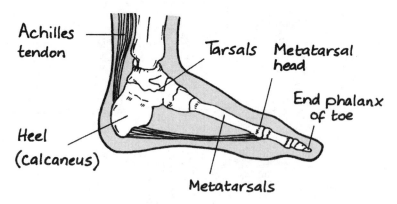

Side View of Foot

Achilles tendon

Tarsals

Metatarsal head

End phalanx of toe

Heel (calcaneus)

Metatarsals

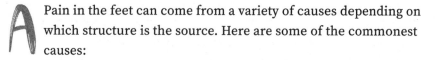

Q Why do my feet hurt when I run?

A Pain in the feet can come from a variety of causes depending on which structure is the source. Here are some of the commonest causes:

- **Muscular pain** Pain from strained or over-worked muscles. It's common if you're building up distance, running on uneven ground or in the wrong shoes. Pain and tenderness is usually felt over the affected muscle, and pain is aggravated by using and stretching the muscle.
- **Plantar fasciitis** Pain in the heel and sole of the foot (see page 156).
- **Tendonitis** Pain from inflamed or strained tendons from over use or injury. Pain at the back of the foot may be due to Achilles tendonitis. The tendons running just below the knobbly bits on the inside and outside of the ankle (medial and lateral malleoli) are common sites too, resulting in pain in the side of the foot arch where they attach to the foot bones.
- **Metatarsalgia** Pain in the heads of the metatarsal bones. Felt in the ball of the foot, this may give the sensation of standing on

a pebble, and is usually due to increased intensity and volume of running. There are multiple other causes, including obesity, high-heeled shoes and arthritis.

- **Morton's Neuroma** Another cause of metatarsalgia. This is common in runners (see page 158).
- **Nerve pain** A compressed nerve can cause pain, tingling and numbness. Nerves can be trapped, irritated or over-stretched at any point along their journey from the spine to the foot, so even if the pain is felt in the foot, the problem could be in the back. This is often painful at rest.
- **Stress fracture** An over-use injury, stress fractures are more likely in those who have osteoporosis (low bone density). They tend to occur in the metatarsal or calcaneus bones of the feet. They require prolonged periods of rest and a gradual return to running (see page 150).
- **Arthritis** A 'wear and tear' arthritis or a more aggressive arthritis such as rheumatoid arthritis can affect foot bones. Pain, stiffness and swelling result from loss of cushioning cartilage. It's still important to exercise as much as you are able to (see page 144).

Clearly, differentiating between all of these can be tricky and foot pain can take time to diagnose. If you're unsure, then try a brief period of rest and a gentle return to activity. If your pain persists, seek a diagnosis from a health care professional.

Foot-strengthening exercises

TRY THIS AT HOME

Often you don't need support in your running shoes, you just need stronger feet! Here are four simple things you can do to improve your foot strength:

1. Walk barefoot whenever you get the chance.
2. While sitting on a chair, put both feet on the floor (barefoot is best). Raise your heels, keeping the ball of both feet on the ground. Hold for five seconds. Then raise the ball off

continued overleaf ▶

so your weight is just on the tips of your toes. Hold for five seconds. Slowly lower your foot, working back through the toes and the ball of the foot on the way down. Repeat ten times.

3 While sitting at your desk, place both feet on the ground and scrunch your feet up, drawing your toes in and foot arch off the floor. Hold for five seconds then relax. Repeat ten times.

4 Sitting or standing, put a large piece of paper or tissue on the floor. Place your bare foot on it, and try to grip the paper and lift it off the ground. Place it back down again. Repeat ten times.

Q I've been told I have plantar fasciitis. What exactly is it and do I have to stop running?

A Under the skin on the sole of your feet there's a tough connective tissue, extending from the heel bones right up to near the base of the toes, called the plantar fascia. When you add 'itis' on to anything in medicine it means inflammation, but we no longer think that much inflammation is involved in plantar fasciitis (PF) beyond the early stages of the condition. The plantar fascia helps to support the arch of the foot and absorbs some of the force when the foot strikes the ground. Acting almost like an elastic tissue, the fascia turns strain into propulsive energy, pushing you forwards as the tension is released when the foot leaves the ground.

We don't understand why PF happens. It has been thought to be due to the force of landing, but that doesn't explain why people with sedentary lifestyles suffer from it too. Studies looking at the relationship between PF and the Achilles tendon show that when PF is present, the Achilles is often thickened and the muscles at the back of the leg are often tight. This is a bit of a chicken and egg situation, because we don't know which came first. It seems to happen in runners who increase their distance or intensity of training rapidly, so beginners often get it. It's almost certainly linked to running biomechanics, possibly the strength of your foot arch, how your foot hits the ground, your shoes and a host of other factors that are very individual.

When you get PF it becomes painful to put your foot on the ground – or you might be unlucky and have both feet affected at the same time. Pain is usually felt around the heel, especially when you first get out of bed in the morning and when walking barefoot. Initially the pain eases up with gentle walking, but sometimes PF progresses until it's felt continuously.

So, what can you do about it? PF usually goes away eventually, but it can take six months to a year. It's best to rest initially and let any inflammation settle down. Avoid doing anything that aggravates the pain. You'll probably have to stop running but if running isn't making it hurt then there's no real reason not to carry on. You can use ice packs and anti-inflammatories such as ibuprofen in a gel or tablet form. Heel pads can take the pressure off the fascia and choose whichever shoes feel most comfortable.

Stretch out the fascia by doing exercises such as sitting with your legs outstretched in front of you and using a scarf looped around the ball of your foot to bring your foot towards you. Rolling a frozen water bottle or a golf ball under your foot can give relief too. Because of the link with the calves and Achilles, it's a good idea to do stretches that lengthen your calf muscles. An assessment by a physiotherapist will help identify any specific triggers from your own biomechanics. Other possible treatments include steroid injections, night splints such as the Strassburg Sock, which keeps your foot flexed and stretched while you sleep, and Extracorporeal Shock Wave Therapy, where low-energy sound waves are passed through the skin to the injured area of the foot in order to increase blood flow and speed up the healing process. However, results can be very varied. Go back to running gradually, when you're pain free, and continue with the stretches to help keep it at bay.

Q My GP thinks I have a Morton's Neuroma. Has running caused this?

A Morton's Neuroma is one of many causes of metatarsalgia (pain in the metatarsals). It's caused by thickening of one of the nerves that run between the metatarsal bones, usually the second, third or fourth metatarsals. Pain, tingling or numbness can be felt in the area of the affected nerve and people say it feels like there's a pebble under the ball of their foot when they walk. It usually presents in one foot, around age 50, and is more common in women than men. Runners are at high risk of a Morton's Neuroma due to compression and irritation of the nerve when the feet repeatedly strike the ground. The pain can come and go or be continuous. One third of people get better with rest, comfortable footwear and metatarsal pads inserted into shoes (these are available to buy over the counter). Steroid and local anaesthetic injections can help relieve symptoms and there are surgical procedures to cut out or make more room for (decompress) the nerve if symptoms are ongoing.

Q Which part of my foot should I land on when I run?

A The issue of how your foot should strike the ground when you run is a very controversial one. There are essentially three options: forefoot, midfoot and hindfoot. With a forefoot strike you land on your toes and ball of your foot. Midfoot means landing on the centre of your foot (your heel and ball of the foot strike the ground simultaneously) and with a hindfoot technique your heel strikes the ground first. Start observing people's feet and you will see runners using all three of these landings. Beginner runners and those who run more slowly over longer distances often use the hindfoot landing, also known as heel striking. The faster you run, the more likely it is that you'll have a forefoot landing, it's hard to find a sprinter who heel strikes.

Heel striking has had very bad press and runners (myself included) have been encouraged to move to a midfoot strike. The reasons for this make a great deal of sense to me. With a marked heel strike, when you land you are essentially putting on a brake. Your body weight is behind your foot and you have to overcome that backwards force in order to move forwards. That's not helpful when it comes to running efficiency. The leading leg is outstretched, often with a locked-out knee at the time of impact, putting pressure on the knee joint in a direction that it wasn't designed for. In addition, you can't benefit from the propulsive power of your foot arch to help you spring forwards. Compare this to a midfoot landing where your body weight is directly over your knee as you land, everything is aligned, and the foot arch can then flatten onto the ground and propel you forwards as it shortens when you lift off.

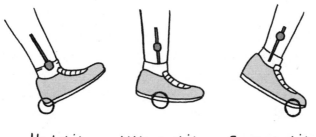

Heel strike   Midfoot strike   Forefoot strike

Heel striking is very common because of our sedentary lifestyle. When we sit for long periods we develop weak glutes and tight hip flexors. Instead of being upright and having our pelvis tucked underneath us when we run, our hips sink down, bottom sticks out and we run as if we're still sitting on a sofa. We run as if we're walking and the two are different. Running is actually jumping, because there's a time when both feet are off the ground.

With a marked forefoot landing, bodyweight is usually ahead of the landing leg. If you take your shoes off and run barefoot you'll probably find that you land on your forefoot or midfoot. Most people do. Many choose to run barefoot or in very minimalist shoes, believing we're designed to run barefoot, and because they have found they have fewer injuries and better running performance. However, while heel striking can lead to knee injury, there's significant concern that a strong forefoot landing leads to more Achilles injuries. If you watch someone who is purely forefoot running, you'll observe that their calf is continuously under tension and it's easy to see how that can lead to Achilles tendon problems.

Did you know?

There are 28 bones and over 100 ligaments in each of your feet.

Q Should I try to change my foot strike?

A Some people argue that, no, you shouldn't. Everyone is different and just do what comes naturally. Some running is better than no running, regardless of how you land. To a certain extent I agree and I certainly wouldn't advocate changing your foot strike yourself without the advice of an experienced running coach. It should only ever be done very gradually and it can take years for it to become natural. However, if you have certain issues or injuries, want to address a plateau in your running speed or just feel that your running isn't optimal, then it's worth seeing a running coach who has experience in running gait. There are other simpler things they may suggest prior to focusing purely on your feet, including improving your posture, shortening your stride and increasing your running cadence. These in themselves may be enough to give you the outcomes you want. All of these will most likely encourage your body away from a heel strike and towards a midfoot strike. In the meantime, I continue my personal endeavour to master a subconscious midfoot strike.

Q I've got pain at the back of my ankle. Is it my Achilles and can I carry on running?

A This could well be pain from your Achilles tendon as it's a fairly frequent problem in runners. You need to be a bit careful here, because ignoring it and just carrying on running risks long-term damage. The Achilles tendon connects your calf muscles (the gastrocnemius and soleus) to your heel bone (the calcaneus). When the calf muscles contract, the tendon helps to lift the heel off the ground. Running can put a lot of stress on the Achilles, particularly if you increase your frequency or distance of running too quickly, and if you do a lot of hill running or speed work. You might have heard of Achilles tendonitis, which was thought to be a simple inflammation of the tendon from over use, but we now know that although there may be some initial inflammatory changes, over time, microscopic injury, including tears, occur in the individual tendon fibres. The tendon may thicken and become stiffer to protect itself. This is more accurately called Achilles tendinopathy. The structure and strength of the tendon is altered, and if ignored then it can ultimately lead to weakening and, at worst, complete rupture (tearing) of the Achilles.

Don't ignore Achilles pain, swelling, thickening or lumps. Taking early action can prevent a lengthy recovery, prolonged time off running or a potential tendon rupture. First you should rest to take the strain off the Achilles. Apply ice (15 minutes several times a day), gently massage or foam roll your calf muscles to relax them and consider taking an anti-inflammatory. This should help to ease the initial symptoms, but you then need to move onto a longer-term strategy to strengthen your calf muscles and look for underlying causes. If it was simply increasing your distance too quickly, then a period of rest and a gradual return to running with adequate rest days may suffice, but it may be more complicated than this. Poor biomechanics, muscle imbalances, tightness and weakness can all lead to Achilles problems. This is a specialist area and I highly advise seeing a physiotherapist who can tailor a recovery programme to your exact situation. With careful management you can avoid or at least reduce your chances of long-term Achilles problems.

Real-life runners

My Achilles issues were improved by getting some professional help from a specialist chiropractor. She taught me great stretching techniques and, being a runner herself, understood the mental side too – the drive to have to run! Following her advice, learning techniques to improve my stability and mobility, plus my investment in some compression socks, has really helped.

Mike Whelan, runner and Leinster Rugby fanatic

Q I've sprained my ankle. What's the best way for me to get back to running as quickly as possible?

A Don't underestimate the common sprained ankle. Even though no bones have been broken, a sprain can cause significant problems. Ligaments stabilise joints and when sprained they get overstretched and torn, for example by going over on your ankle. The pain, swelling and any instability of the joint needs careful management to get you back running as soon as possible. Good rehabilitation of ankle injuries is crucial if you want to return to full strength.

Use the PRICE protocol (see page 209) as first-aid for your ankle and assess how severe your injury is. If there's no swelling, and you can still weight-bear without too much difficulty, then you've got a minor sprain and might be running again after two weeks. If the pain or swelling is immediately very severe, or you're still unable to weight-bear after two days of PRICE, then you need to be medically assessed in case you have broken a bone. Assuming no fracture is seen, then it's a case of working hard and being very patient, because severe sprains can mean four to six months off running.

Rehabilitation focuses on getting flexibility, strength and stability back in your ankle. It's best to be up and about, gently mobilising, as soon as you can. In the first couple of days start by gently flexing and extending your ankle several times through the day. Try using a towel looped under your foot to gently pull it towards you. Build up to rotating it and writing the alphabet in the air with your foot by the end of the first week. Then you can start to do some strength work, gently pushing your foot into the ground, aiming to be able to stand on one leg. Try going up and down on your toes (calf raises), with both feet at once in the early stages. You can do this sitting in a chair if standing is too hard initially. Once you feel confident and strong with up and down movements, then add in some sideways and twisting ones, such as standing on one leg while twisting your body, side stepping and walking in a figure of eight. If at any point your ankle begins to swell more then it's a sign that you're doing too much. Elevate it, reduce your activities and then slowly build up again. You may want to invest in an ankle support or get a physiotherapist to advise you how to tape your ankle.

The point at which you can run will depend hugely on the individual, but once you feel confident with the stability, strength and flexibility of your ankle then you can begin to jog and then run. Start on a treadmill or find some flat grass – avoid uneven and bumpy surfaces. In reality it takes around 12 weeks for ligaments to heal up, so even if you feel OK, do take care for three or four months.

HIPS AND SPINE

Q I've heard other runners talk about piriformis syndrome. What is it?

A Piriformis syndrome is quite literally a pain in the bum! The piriformis is a muscle which runs from your lower spine (sacrum) out to the top of your thigh bone. It's located behind the gluteus maximum muscle, but is much smaller than this giant. You have one on each side of your body and its job is to help rotate the hip and turn your legs outwards. If the muscle becomes tight, swollen or spasms, then you can get buttock pain. You might also get pain down the back of your leg and tingling or numbness due to irritation of your sciatic nerve, which runs close to the piriformis. The pain can be worse if you've been sitting for a while and it can also be triggered by running, particularly uphill, and going up stairs. We don't really know why it happens, but prolonged sitting is certainly a risk factor. Treatment focuses on stretching out the piriformis. You can do these lying or seated.

Piriformis Stretches

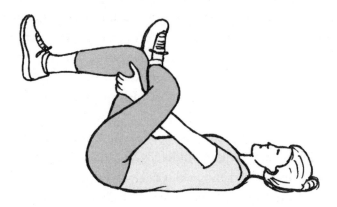

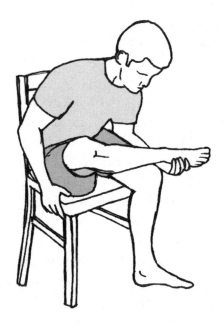

You may need input from a physiotherapist if simple home stretches aren't enough to ease your symptoms.

Q Can I run with sciatica?

A No. To understand this answer, it helps to know exactly what sciatica is. Running irritates sciatica, but it doesn't directly cause it. The sciatic nerve comes out from the lower part of the spinal cord and travels down through the buttock, down the back of the thigh to the calf and under the foot. When it is squashed it causes pain, tingling, numbness and occasionally weakness in the area below the compression. It most commonly becomes compressed at the spine by a 'slipped disc'. Discs are basically gel pads acting as shock absorbers between each of our vertebrae (back bones). When a disc 'slips', some of the disc bulges out (prolapses) and compresses the nerves at their root. This can then cause symptoms anywhere along the nerve. Remember, the sciatic nerve can be compressed by the piriformis muscle too. Sciatica tends to cause a pain in the buttock and down the back of the thigh, but it can extend down to the lower leg and under the sole of the foot, and be associated with reduced sensation and tingling.

Knowing this, it's easy to see why running is not a good idea if you have sciatica from a prolapsed disc. The impact of running will put extra stress onto the bulging disc and further compress the sciatic nerve. It's not all bad news, though, because not all cases of sciatica are from prolapsed discs. Most will resolve and we know that generally being active helps to prevent back pain. Plenty of runners have had sciatica in the past and are no longer bothered by it. What is crucial is that you don't try to run through any pain and you allow long enough for the sciatica to settle (four to six weeks). A physiotherapist to identify the cause of your sciatic nerve irritation, and help you properly rehabilitate and return to running gradually, is invaluable.

Q Why does running give me pain in the back of my neck?

A Do you wake up the day after a long run with pain and stiffness in the back of your neck? This is another perfect example of how what goes on in one part of your body affects another. Running is a high-impact activity and pain in your neck suggests that your running posture isn't ideal. Sometimes the pain is purely muscular, but it may also be from the cervical spine (neck bones) and surrounding structures. It suggests that the way you are landing when you run is placing excess stress on your neck. This is most prevalent in people who run with a marked heel strike. Working on your running posture should help. If your pain is persistent, not purely caused by running, or you have symptoms such as numbness or tingling in your arms, then see your GP for an assessment.

Running posture tips

Running with good posture will help to minimise your risk of injury, improve your running technique and make you a more efficient runner. Try the following tips. You could focus on one each time you run until you have mastered them all:

- Stand up tall.
- Make sure your shoulders are back.
- Hold your head up high.
- Engage your core muscles.
- Tuck your bottom under.
- Keep your hips strong and level when you run.
- Lean forwards slightly from your ankles not your hips.
- Don't over stride. Try to land with your body balanced directly over your foot.
- Let your arms swing in a forward and back motion, at your side and close to your body.

Q Why do lots of runners get ITB problems?

A Most runners will have heard of the iliotibial band (ITB) as it's frequently blamed for injuries and discomfort. It's a thick band of dense tissue, which runs from the ileum bone in the pelvis down the outer thigh to the outside of the knee, where it attaches to the tibia bone below the knee cap. It helps to stabilise the hip and knee, and works with the hip muscles during movement. Pain from the ITB can be felt anywhere along its route, but is most commonly felt at the side of the knee. Iliotibial band syndrome (ITBS) is experienced by up to 14 per cent of runners, with the highest risk groups being those who are increasing their distance, running high mileage and those with biomechanical issues. The pain tends to come on at about the same distance each time you run and is often worse when running downhill.

The exact cause of the pain and the treatment for ITBS is actually poorly understood, with limited evidence to back up theories and treatment plans. It's probably more complex than simple friction and inflammation of the band. It's more likely to happen if you have weak hip muscles, a tight ITB or an uneven running style. It's thought that women may be affected more than men because their wider pelvis and the angle of their thigh bones puts the ITB under more tension.

Thankfully ITBS usually resolves. Around half of runners will be back running after eight weeks and only 10 per cent will still be off running after six months. When it first happens you should reduce or change your activities. Don't do anything that causes you pain, which means you will probably have to stop running and switch to swimming or walking for a few weeks. There is some controversy over whether stretching or massaging your ITB (including with a foam roller) will help. Try stretching your ITB with a banana stretch to see if it gives you any relief. Cross your affected leg behind your healthy one while standing up tall and, with your arms raised above your head, lean away from the affected leg to make yourself into a banana shape. You should feel the stretch right up the outside of your hip, thigh and knee.

Like most running injuries it's important to correct any underlying cause, so look for exercises that you can do regularly to help build up strength in your hip muscles. Resistance bands are perfect for this and a few minutes every day using a band will be time well spent.

You can gradually build up your running distance again, but keep going with the strength exercises. Listen to your body. If you feel your ITB start to twinge then cut down again. If you think it's more than just a case of running too much too soon, get a gait analysis to make sure you have the right shoes, and if you have recurrent ITBS, then see a physiotherapist for an assessment.

Real-life runners

At the beginning of my running journey, I had ITB issues. After
a lot of research and seeing a running physio, I discovered
I had weak glutes and weak foot arches. Initially I tried custom-
made insoles but they seemed to cause more problems and
didn't correct the root cause. Doing specific strength exercises
focusing on my glutes, core and foot strength gradually started
to pay off, and over time I found my gait changed and my pain
disappeared.

Lisa Ruggles, runner, coach and director of 261 Fearless Club UK CIC

Q My knees are fine, but running seems to cause pain in my hips. What could this be?

A This could be Greater Trochanteric Pain Syndrome (GTPS), which
can often afflict women who are between 40 and 50. Pain is felt
in the outside of the hip. It's worse when you lie on it, cross
your legs or do repetitive movements, such as walking, cycling or
running. You might have heard it called trochanteric bursitis, because
it was thought to be due to inflammation of the bursa or fluid-filled
cushions around the greater trochanter, a large bump at the top of the
thigh bone. We now know that it isn't as straightforward as this and
likely involves small injuries to the muscles and tendons around the
trochanter too. While also being caused by being overweight and sitting
for too long (particularly with crossed legs), the repetitive movement of
running is a clear trigger and runners who are rapidly increasing their
distance are at particular risk.

Treatment involves a period off running, usually a few weeks,
to let any inflammation settle. Try to keep doing light exercise and
stick to your normal daily routine during this. You may need to
use some painkillers such as paracetamol and you can apply ice
to the sore, tender areas. Follow this with strengthening exercises

to address any weaknesses in hip and thigh muscles, and follow that with a gradual return to running. Exercises can include glute bridges, single leg stands, wall squats and hip abduction exercises, which involve keeping your pelvis still and moving your leg sideways away from your body. You can use a resistance band for this movement too.

If your pain is not settling, then sometimes corticosteroid injections are used and you should see a physiotherapist or doctor to check the diagnosis and discuss further options.

TOP TIPS FOR A HEALTHY RUNNER'S MUSCULOSKELETAL SYSTEM

The musculoskeletal system can seem complicated and overwhelming, but there are some simple things you can do to help keep yours in good shape for many happy running miles:

- Always increase the volume and intensity of training gradually.
- Allow enough recovery days.
- Wear correct footwear, professionally fitted if possible.
- Use strength and conditioning to give you a strong and balanced body.
- Be aware that strength and balance training become more important as you age.
- Warm up with dynamic stretches rather than static ones, which should be done after a cool-down.
- See a health care professional for a diagnosis if any pain is not resolving.
- Maintain a healthy weight.
- Eat a balanced and varied diet so your body has the building blocks it needs for growth and repair.
- Find a good physiotherapist who is experienced in helping runners – they're worth their weight in gold.

FURTHER HELP AND ADVICE

Royal Osteoporosis Society: www.theros.org.uk
Versus Arthritis: www.versusarthritis.org
Running Physio: www.running-physio.com
General advice on conditions: www.patient.info
Find a physio – Chartered Society of Physiotherapy: www.csp.org.
   uk/public-patient/find-physiotherapist/physio2u

CHAPTER 8

....

THE SKIN

If you could design the ultimate running kit it would be comfortable, waterproof, breathable, both warm and cool, fit snuggly and stretch when you need it to. Skin is perfectly designed for use during running, given it meets all of these criteria and has many more functions too! Despite this, though, there are issues that crop up and problems that arise with your skin that can be minor inconveniences or total game-changers, preventing you from taking even a single step. Let's look at the body's largest organ, learn more about how it works and what we can do to look after our most precious running kit.

Skin is incredibly clever! Here's a list of just some of the roles that skin has:

- Holds us together.
- Protects the tissues that lie underneath.
- Controls body temperature.
- Keeps out infection.
- Prevents damage from ultraviolet light.
- Gets rid of toxins.
- Allows us to touch and feel.
- Makes vitamin D.
- Allows movement.

There are three main layers to the skin: the epidermis, the dermis and the hypodermis.

The Skin

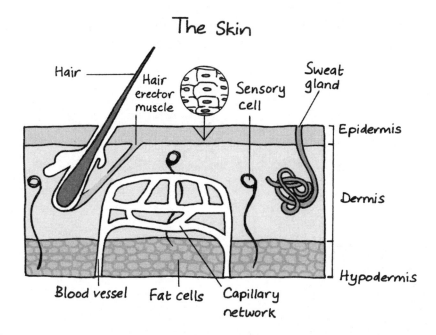

The epidermis is at the surface and is made up of layers of epithelial cells. Where your skin is thin, for example on your eyelids, there will be fewer layers than where it's thick, on the soles of your feet and palms of your hands. The top layer of epithelial cells dies and sheds continuously, and is replaced by newer cells moving up from the deeper layers. Skin pigment cells called melanocytes are found in the deep layers of the epidermis.

The dermis is a much thicker layer and contains sweat glands, nerve fibres, blood vessels, hair follicles and defence cells to prevent infection. These structures are all held together by a mesh of connective tissue containing collagen and elastin fibres, to give it both strength and stretch.

The hypodermis is also called the subcutaneous layer and is largely made up of fatty tissue called adipose tissue. It's not strictly part of the skin, but it links the skin to underlying muscles and bones, supports the skin's structures and provides an insulating, cushioned layer that is important for temperature regulation and protection.

Once you've got your head around basic skin anatomy and function, it not only gives you great respect for it and an appreciation of its complexity, but also a good base to work from when trying to understand and solve running-related skin issues. Let's move on to some frequently asked questions, starting with skin damage and moving on to infections, followed by long-term skin conditions.

SKIN TRAUMA AND DAMAGE

Q How can I stop my skin chafing on long runs?

A Sometimes you can grin and bear a bit of chafing when you run, but when you get in the shower afterwards, even the faintest red patches can cause searing pain! Chafing is caused either by skin rubbing against skin, such as between your thighs, or fabric rubbing against skin, such as under bra straps or waist bands. Adding in the dampness caused by sweat is a recipe for chafing. Skin sheds its top layer of epithelial cells naturally, but when friction and rubbing accelerate this loss, then lower layers of cells become exposed. These cells are not designed to be, or haven't matured enough to be, on the outside. Nerve endings and small blood vessels are exposed and surrounding skin gets angry and inflamed too. Chafing can be treated, but the best bet is prevention.

Well-fitting clothes in the right fabrics will make a big difference. There's a reason why runners wear Lycra! Close-fitting kit that sits snug to the skin tends to rub less than baggier clothes which move around more. Lycra shorts or leggings will stop thighs rubbing against each other, because, let's face it, how many of us actually have a thigh gap? Many men however report they chafe less in loose fitting shorts so it can be trial and error. Sports bras can be trickier as there's a lot of natural movement (see page 176), but the best fit possible with soft, seam-free fabrics generally helps. Wet clothes rub most so choose a fabric which wicks well – this means it draws sweat away from the body and dries quickly.

For problem areas which always seem to rub, apply a skin-protecting lubricant before running to add an extra layer. This is especially useful if you're going to get wet. In sweaty areas, you can also try using your antiperspirant.

Treating chafed skin

TRY THIS AT HOME

If, despite your best efforts, you find yourself with an area of sore, inflamed skin, here's what to do:

1. Clean the area thoroughly with warm water and a mild soap. Avoid anything too strong or perfumed.
2. Pat the skin dry with a soft, clean towel.
3. Apply a soothing antiseptic cream or protective balm. Nappy creams that contain zinc oxide are ideal.
4. If possible, allow the skin to be exposed to the air. Baggy clothes are best.
5. Protect the skin from further damage. This may mean covering it with a sterile dressing to stop it sticking to clothes or getting rubbed again.
6. Skin will heal in a few days. While a bit of itching is normal, watch for signs of infection, including a sticky discharge, an unpleasant odour and increasing redness around the wound.

Q No matter what I try, on my longest runs my nipples always end up really sore and bleeding. What can I do?

A Runner's nipple is common in men because of friction between t-shirts and protruding nipples. It's less common in women due to sports bras acting as a barrier. Try following the advice above about chafing. You might find that a very close-fitting base layer that clings to your chest like a second skin will help. If you feel self-conscious wearing one, then choose a vest style and wear a t-shirt over the top. Protective lubricant is essential and consider putting a small pot in your running belt so you can re-apply mid-run. If you're still struggling, then you can stick tape, plasters or pads over your nipples to protect them. There are a variety of products available, from basic surgical tape to specially designed nipple pads for runners. It's always difficult to guarantee they'll remain in place, particularly if you sweat heavily, and they can be painful to remove from hairy chests but they're certainly worth a try. If you're a new runner, you'll probably find your nipples toughen up with time.

Real-life runners

My nipples started chafing and bleeding when my runs increased in length and frequency. This didn't bother me too much when I was running, but afterwards in the shower the water on the broken skin was painful. Sports lubricant only worked on short runs. The solution for me was tape. I just had to make sure it was the right length, so it didn't stick to my chest hair and fall off.

Jason Redman, marathon runner in training

Q How can I take care of my breasts when I run? I'm worried running will make them sag.

A Whether you are breast feeding or not, and regardless of your age, it's important to look after your breasts when you run. Breasts are made of fatty tissue held in place by underlying muscles, overlying skin and a network of fibres called Cooper's ligaments. Breast-sagging is largely determined by your genetics and how elastic your tissues are rather than by how much you run. Breasts move in a figure of eight motion during running and can move up to 10 centimetres. It's important to reduce this movement as much as possible to prevent the ligaments becoming overstretched. A good sports bra is the best way to do this and it is worth investing time and money to find the right one for you. Women usually wear a chest band that is too loose and cup size that is too small. If possible, find a shop with an experienced bra fitter and variety of bras you can try on. Many online stores have free returns so you can order different styles and sizes, and send back what you don't need. The bigger your breasts, the more support you will need. Opt for wide shoulder straps to distribute weight and a mix of compression to squash your breasts against your chest wall and encapsulation to support each breast individually. Don't forget that bras wear out and lose their elastic support, so if you can't remember how old yours is it probably needs replacing!

Did you know?

It's quite a shocking statistic, but 70 per cent of women wear a bra that is the wrong size for them.

Q I get chilblains every winter. Will running help them or make them worse?

A We don't really know why some people get chilblains and others don't, but these red or purple lumps can be itchy and painful. They develop in response to the cold and are more common on extremities such as toes and fingers, but you can also get them on ears, noses, cheeks and even your legs. Anyone can get them, but people who have poor circulation, who smoke or have diabetes, tend to get them more often. They are also more likely to develop if you warm up cold skin too quickly, by putting your feet on the radiator or plunging your hands into hot water, for example. The good news is that they usually go away by themselves, within a couple of weeks. No treatment is necessary other than keeping them warm. Running may be triggering them if you're out in cold weather and re-warming too quickly. Layer up to keep your body warm and invest in warm socks (merino wool is ideal) and well-insulated gloves. Exercise does, however, boost circulation generally and you may just be someone who is prone to chilblains. They often run in the family. They can be a pain, but aren't harmful and you can generally keep running.

Did you know?

Double dipping, where you take some lubricant from a communal pot and apply it to your body and then put your fingers back in to take some more, is illegal. Well, actually it's not, but it should be! Use a spoon or wooden spatula to take out what you need to prevent germs growing in the lubricant. Please don't double dip!

Q I get huge blisters. What can I do to prevent them?

A Blisters form in or just under the epidermis. Friction and resulting skin damage from rubbing shoes and socks is the commonest cause for runners, but extreme cold, heat, chemical damage and medical conditions can all cause blisters too. Fluid (serum) fills the damaged space to protect the tissues underneath. The fluid is usually clear, it may be bloodstained if it's a blood blister or, if the blister is infected, the fluid may be a thicker, discoloured pus. They're incredibly common and annoying, but here are some things you can do to try to prevent them:

- **Get the right shoes.** Go up at least half a size from your normal shoe to make sure there's enough space for your feet to spread and swell a little when you run. Wear new shoes in before you hit the big miles.
- **Learn to lace.** Everyone's feet are different and you can help problem areas by altering your lacing. There are different lacing techniques for issues such as a wide forefoot or a high instep (see page 153).
- **Don't forget your socks.** The right socks are crucial for blister prevention and it can be a case of trial and error, with some runners favouring single layer socks and others double layer. A technical fabric that wicks away sweat and dries quickly will keep feet dry. Wet fabric and wet feet makes blisters more likely.
- **Use a barrier.** You can apply some lubricant to your skin to help protect it, or try a talcum powder if you think sweaty feet are a cause for you. Plasters tend to move or fall off and you may have more luck with specially designed blister tape.
- **Avoid chemicals to toughen your feet.** By all means steer clear of the moisturiser and allow your feet to naturally toughen, but I'd advise against using alcohol or surgical spirit to speed up the process. You often end up with painful cracks and fissures which cause their own problems.

Real-life runners

I used to get terrible blisters, usually between my toes and on the balls of my feet, despite loads of lube before marathons. Strangely, though, once I stopped using it I had far fewer problems. I think the lube was just making my feet slide around in my shoe. I hardly get them now.

Tara Cunnington, runs, sings and dances

Q What's the best way to treat my blisters? Is it OK to pop them?

A I don't recommend popping blisters. Even the tiniest hole can be a route in for infection. While the skin is intact the contents of the blister are sterile. The fluid is also acting as a cushion to protect the delicate skin beneath. If you're mid-ultra and absolutely need to pop them to be able to continue, then the ideal technique would be to use a sterile needle and syringe to aspirate (draw out) the fluid. If this isn't possible then use a sterile needle to make a small hole and gently milk it out. Follow with a sterile dressing and tape it down firmly. If you're not popping or your blister has popped on its own, then the goal is to keep it clean, dry and cushioned. Warm soapy water is adequate to clean it. Pat it dry and then apply a padded dressing. I like the hydrocolloid ones. Small blisters will shrivel up on their own within a few days; larger ones may take a couple of weeks. See your pharmacist or GP if you think your blister is infected – there may be redness which is spreading further and further out from the blister or it may be filled with pus.

Heel lock

TRY THIS AT HOME

One cause of blisters is your feet moving around too much inside your shoe. If you have a narrow heel and ankle and your feet aren't secured properly, then this can create a lot of movement. You might find your toes hit the end of your shoes during downhill running when your feet slip forward. This can cause toenail damage as well as heel blisters. The handy 'heel lock' is a trick that many runners don't know about – it's why there is that extra hole for lacing at the top of your shoe which is usually ignored!

Lace your shoes up in a criss-cross pattern, finishing with the laces coming out of the shoes in the top hole.

continued overleaf ▶

2　Create a loop by taking the lace and threading it back in towards the shoe through that second spare eyelet on the same side.

3　Cross the laces and pass them through the loop on the opposite side, from inside to outside.

4　Pull the laces tight to lock the heel in place and tie the laces as normal.

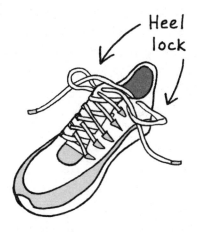

Heel lock

Q Is being outside a lot damaging my skin? How can I protect it and what signs of damage do I need to look out for?

A It's a good idea to protect your skin from ultraviolet rays as much as you can when you run, especially on sunny days. You can do this by wearing a good sunscreen (at least SPF 15), a cap or visor, and covering your shoulders and arms if you're going to be out for some time. Wear good quality sunglasses to protect your eyes. Runners often complain that sunscreen slides off when they sweat and ends up stinging their eyes, but there are many sweat-resistant ones available. Remember that you can still burn on cloudy days.

The first sign of damage is an obvious one – sunburn. Don't be the runner who forgot to put cream on before their marathon and has painful sunburn as well as DOMS to deal with! Ultraviolet radiation damages skin cells. The skin tries to limit damage and begin repair by dilating blood vessels to increase circulation to the area. That's why skin turns red when it's burnt. The skin then dries out and eventually the top layers peel off. The DNA of skin cells can be harmed and altered by ultraviolet rays, potentially leading to skin cancer.

Another sign of damage is changing moles. Any mole which is growing in size or thickness, bleeds, itches or crusts, needs to be checked by a doctor. So do moles that are becoming darker, changing shape or appear to be spreading outwards into the surrounding skin. These are all potential red flags for the serious skin cancer melanoma, so don't put off getting checked. You can take a photo on your phone of any moles you're unsure of so you can see if they're changing.

You may not have heard of actinic keratoses (also called solar keratoses). These develop over many years of sun exposure and are more common if you're over 50. You might notice a dry, rough or scaly patch in areas such as the face, forearms or on a bald head. They vary in colour from a pale pink skin colour to deeper red and often have a white, crusty scale on the top. Actinic keratoses aren't actually harmful and will often go away on their own, but because there's a small risk they can turn into a type of skin cancer, called a squamous cell carcinoma (SCC), they're usually treated. Treatment may involve freezing them off, applying cream or having the patches scraped away.

Finally, older runners should be aware of basal cell carcinoma (BCC), another non-melanoma skin cancer that is related to sun exposure. Lesions are usually on the head and neck and more common in men than women. BCCs tend to start as a small, painless lump, just a few millimetres across, which is either pink or pearly coloured, and grows very slowly over months. Sometimes they can bleed, develop a crust or ulcerate. BCCs rarely metastasise – spread to other places in the body – so treatment is not as urgent as for a melanoma.

In summary, because of potential high sun exposure, it's wise to take steps to protect your skin, be skin aware, check moles regularly and see your doctor about any skin lesions you are unsure of.

Q Will running make my face sag?

A It's not unreasonable to think that the repetitive up and down movement of running might make your face sag, but there's no evidence that runners have more droopy or wrinkled skin than non-runners. In fact, exercise can be anti-ageing (see page 221). It's largely your genetics that determine the elasticity of your skin and how ready it is to bounce back after gravity has pulled it down. Ultraviolet rays will decrease the skin's elastic properties, so follow the advice above about protecting your skin from the sun. If you use a daily moisturiser on your face, consider one that contains an SPF so you always have a degree of protection when you're running outside.

SKIN INFECTIONS

Q I keep getting athlete's foot. It seems to clear up and then just comes back again. What can I do?

A Athlete's foot is a fungal infection. Fungi love damp, warm, dark places, so where better than a runner's sweaty shoe? It's also known as tinea pedis, with 'tinea' meaning fungus and 'pedis' meaning foot. It can affect your skin in a number of ways. It may become dry and cracked or moist and split, especially between or under the toes. It can look white or red, it may peel or bleed, feel sore or painful, and it's often itchy – sometimes intensely so. You can treat it with anti-fungal creams, sprays and powders from your local pharmacy.

Examples of anti-fungal medications include terbinafine, miconazole and clotrimazole. Tea-tree oil is often suggested as an alternative treatment, although studies have shown mixed results. Don't apply tea-tree oil directly to skin, dilute it in a carrier oil first and always carry out a small patch test to check for any reactions. If your athlete's foot is very itchy then your pharmacist may suggest a product that has a small amount of hydrocortisone in it to ease the itch. Wash and carefully dry your feet twice a day and after running. Take care to dry thoroughly between your toes with a clean towel. Apply your chosen treatment and then put on clean socks or spend some time barefoot. It's important to continue treating it for a few days after you think it has cleared, just to be on the safe side. If you run daily, then it might be worth having a second pair of running shoes and alternating so they have time to dry out properly. Never be tempted to wear running socks twice. If it really won't budge, then see your GP who may take skin scrapings to confirm the diagnosis and will consider an oral anti-fungal medication to attack the infection from the inside out.

Q I've been looking online and think I might have ring worm in my groin. Do I need to go the doctor?

A Tinea cruris, is the medical term for a fungal infection in the groin. In men it's often called jock itch. Jock is the slang term for American college athletes and the warm sweaty groin of an athlete is the perfect environment for a fungus to grow. It's very similar to athlete's foot (tinea pedis) and it can be the same fungus causing the infection in both areas. This itchy and sometimes sore rash appears on the inner thighs and groin and around the scrotum in men. It is usually pink or red in colour and has an obvious and often slightly raised outline, distinguishing it from neighbouring normal skin. The treatment is the same as for athlete's foot mentioned above. It's crucial to shower straight after exercising to wash away sweat. Then pat the rash dry with a clean towel and lightly apply the anti-fungal cream. Where possible, keep the area exposed to the air rather than covering it. You may find applying a barrier cream before you run will make it more comfortable. You can treat it yourself with advice from the pharmacist. If it isn't clearing, then do see your GP.

Did you know?

Our skin is home to thousands of microorganisms called commensals. They include bacteria, fungi and viruses, and are an important part of the skin microbiota or microbiome, which helps to keep skin infections at bay.

Q I get recurrent thrush. Could it be due to running?

A In the same way that athlete's foot and jock itch fungi can thrive in the warm, moist folds of runners' skin, so can thrush, but thrush is common anyway, so running might not be to blame. Candida albicans is the yeast-like fungus which causes thrush. You might find it under breasts, in armpits or groins. In these locations it's classed as intertrigo, which includes a range of infections and inflammation occurring between skin folds.

The vagina is the commonest site for women to experience thrush. The lining of the vagina and surrounding skin become inflamed, sore and itchy. There's often a white, slightly lumpy vaginal discharge. Men can get thrush on their penis, where redness may develop on head of the penis and foreskin. It can be uncomfortable to pass urine or retract the foreskin and there may be an associated itch and discharge. If you've never had these symptoms before then it's wise to see your GP or go to a sexual health clinic to get the diagnosis confirmed, particularly if you're a man. If you're confident that it's thrush because you've had it before, then you can get treatment from your pharmacist. If the thrush is purely on the skin, then an anti-fungal cream should be effective, but if it's inside the vagina, then a pessary (tablet that is inserted into the vagina) or an oral anti-fungal tablet will be necessary.

Thrush usually clears within a week of treatment, but it has a habit of coming back. To help avoid this you can continue using the cream for a few days after it has seemed to clear. It's also important to avoid things that disrupt the skin's natural bacteria. This is particularly relevant to runners who often shower multiple times a day. Over-washing, especially with strong or perfumed shower gels and soaps, can strip away the healthy bacteria and allow overgrowth of thrush. It's best to avoid these products in sensitive areas and just use water or an emollient soap substitute, such as E45, Oilatum or Doublebase. Make sure skin is completely dry and not left damp. Cotton underwear is better than synthetic materials to avoid recurrent genital thrush. If your thrush isn't clearing or it keeps returning, then do see you GP.

Q I get lots of infected hair follicles in my arm pits. I know sweating when I run isn't helping. What can I do?

The medical term for inflamed or infected hair follicles is folliculitis and it often affects armpits, groins or the beard area. Hair removal by waxing, shaving or plucking makes you more susceptible to folliculitis. It's usually caused by bacteria, particularly staphylococcus aureus, which normally lives harmlessly on the skin. Typically, you'll see red bumps and pustules which can be a bit sore, sometimes mildly itchy, and might weep some clear or pus-coloured discharge. You can try treating it at home by washing the area in salty water or using an antiseptic wash or cream. If this doesn't help, then see your GP who will prescribe an antibiotic cream or tablet. You should generally keep the area as clean and dry as possible, so showering straight after running is important. You can protect sore or inflamed skin while you run by using a barrier cream. Occasionally an infected follicle can turn into a boil or abscess. Top spots for this, especially in active people, are near the anus (perianal abscess) or near the vagina (Bartholin's abscess). These can get extremely painful and you won't be able to run. You might even struggle with walking. See your GP as you will likely need antibiotics and possibly surgical drainage.

Making a salt water soak

TRY THIS AT HOME

With skin conditions you'll often see the advice to 'soak in salty water' to help prevent and treat infections. There's some evidence that plain old water will do just as well, but if you want to try salt water (saline) then it's good to know how to make it yourself. Strong concentrations of salt might aggravate the skin and weak ones will be ineffective. Here's my advice for making a saline soak:

- Use 500 millilitres of warm tap water. If you plan to use this in your nose or eyes, then you should boil it for at least one minute to sterilise it.

continued overleaf ▶

- Add one teaspoon of salt. This can be table salt or fine sea salt (non-iodised).
- Stir until the salt has dissolved.
- Fill a bowl with the salty water and soak the affected area for ten to twenty minutes, twice a day. If this isn't practical, then apply a compress by wetting a clean flannel and pressing it against the inflamed or infected skin.
- Let the area air dry and apply a clean dressing if needed.
- If you want to keep unused solution to use later, then store it in the fridge in a sealed jar that's been washed in hot soapy water. It's best to use it within 24 hours.

Q Any tips for dealing with a verruca? I've got an annoying one on my heel that's a bit sore when I run.

While running itself doesn't put you at high risk of verrucas, your cross training might. They're usually picked up at swimming pools and in communal showers. They are incredibly common and nothing to worry about, but they can occasionally be a bit uncomfortable in your running shoe. Verrucas are basically viral warts on the soles of your feet that grow inwards rather than outwards, due to the fact that you constantly tread on them. You don't actually need to treat them as they will eventually go away on their own, but that can take two years so you need to be patient! There's a strong argument that leaving them to clear is the best option, because it makes you less likely to get another one – your body will have produced the antibodies needed to prevent them. If one is causing you bother and you want to get rid of it, then there are plenty of things you can buy over the counter. Applying salicylic acid to the verruca (avoiding the surrounding skin) and filing away the dead skin the next day is one option. This is very effective, but does take weeks. A quicker option would be to use a home freezing spray. They're expensive and don't work as well as liquid nitrogen, but this is no longer widely available in GP clinics for the treatment of verrucas.

Alternatively, if you want to avoid using chemicals, try duct tape. Stick a piece of tape over the verruca. Take it off every week and soak your foot in warm water for a few minutes. File away the dead skin with an emery board and then reapply the tape. Keep doing this for four weeks. Another natural treatment is to apply a piece of banana skin (soft side down) over the verucca and secure it with a plaster. Do this overnight for two weeks washing the area every morning. The evidence for these methods is variable, but they won't cause any harm and might just do the trick.

Did you know?

When you have diabetes (type 1 or 2), the sensation from the nerves in your feet becomes reduced, so it's easy to get skin sores and blisters and not even know it. If you have diabetes, you should check your feet carefully after each run. Any lesions should be treated promptly because skin healing can be impaired and infections are more likely in diabetics.

SKIN RASHES

Q After I run I get a red, warm, itchy rash on my chest and back. I think it's just heat rash. Can I stop it happening?

A Heat rash is very common, especially if you sweat a lot. Sweat clogs up the pores causing little red spots, which can itch and feel a bit prickly. The best way to prevent it is to keep your skin cool, which is hard if you're a runner. Don't over dress and wear fabrics which wick moisture away from the skin. Keep well hydrated with cold fluids too. It can take a few days to settle and if it's bothering you try applying a cold flannel or ice pack to the skin. Calamine lotion can be soothing, but avoid any perfumed skin creams or washes in case they irritate it. Particularly troublesome heat rash might improve with hydrocortisone cream or antihistamine tablets, but it's best to speak to your pharmacist before you try these and always get confirmation of the diagnosis if things aren't improving.

Q I get these weird blotchy, itchy spots on my skin sometimes, usually after a run or after a post-run shower. They go away the same day, but what are they?

A This sounds like urticaria, the medical term for nettle rash, hives or wheals. The spots are usually pink or white and raised from the skin. They appear in response to a trigger and the number of things that can cause them is huge. Exercise, heat and water appear on this list, all of which may apply to runners! Other causes include stress, certain foods and viral infections. The trigger causes the release of histamine from mast cells in the skin which leads to the rash appearing. If they're mild and disappear within a few hours, then there's no need to treat them. If they're persistent, causing discomfort or continue to spread, then antihistamines will help. If you keep getting urticaria then see your GP to discuss possible causes and treatments. Although rare, if rapidly developing urticaria is associated with lip and tongue swelling or difficulty breathing, then this may indicate a life threatening allergic reaction, called anaphylaxis, and you should dial 999 for an emergency ambulance.

TOENAILS

Q I ran my first marathon a few days ago and three of my toenails have turned black. Do I need to worry?

A There's no need to panic. Black toenails are well known to long distance runners and, while they can look pretty gruesome, they're usually harmless. The black colour is blood from the delicate nail bed that has become trapped under the nail. It's essentially a bruise. The medical term is a subungual haematoma from 'unguis', the Latin word for nail and haematoma, meaning a collection of blood. Don't be alarmed if the nail falls off. This is often inevitable. However, let it stay in place as long as possible so it can protect the nail bed, and don't pull it off. A new nail will gradually grow up from the base, but it may take six to nine months before it's fully grown. Make sure there's enough room for your toes in your running shoes so your nails aren't repeatedly bashing against the end of the shoe, particularly when you run downhill. You might need to go up a full size. Socks which are too small won't help either. Try using the heel lock for lacing your shoes (see page 180) to stop your feet slipping forwards.

Q My big toenail has really thickened up. My GP says it's caused by trauma to the nail, but could it be a fungal infection?

A Both fungal infections and nail trauma can cause a nail to thicken, discolour (usually yellow) and become flaky. It can be hard to tell the difference, but if there is uncertainty scrapings can be taken from the nail and sent to the laboratory for microscopic examination and culture. Even then, the result can be misleading. Fungal infections don't actually need to be treated. There are no serious consequences, but they can spread to other nails. Cosmetically they are unpleasant and the nail can become a bit tender, which makes running hard. If treatment is required, then sadly, there's no quick fix. Although it tends to be the same fungus as athlete's foot that causes nail infections, anti-fungal creams can't penetrate the nail. Either nail lacquers with repeated nail filing or oral antifungal tablets are needed, and these can take six to nine months to work. It's a long process and you should discuss the possible side-effects of anti-fungal tablets, including the risk of liver damage, with your GP. Traumatised nails are more likely to get infected, so make sure your trainers are big enough and practise good foot hygiene to prevent athlete's foot.

Q I keep getting a really sore area on the edge of my big toe, where it meets the nail. Sometimes it weeps and bleeds, and when it's bad I can't run because it's so sore. What can I do?

A This condition is called paronychia, from the Greek 'para' (around) and 'onyx' (nail). It's due to an infection which nestles itself between the skin and the nail. This is more likely to occur if the area has been damaged, which can happen to toenails with the repetitive impact of running, as well as by ingrown nails. When it happens suddenly, it's usually caused by bacteria – staphylococcus aureus is the usual culprit. Redness and swelling develop in the skin alongside the nail and there's often a collection of pus under the skin. This type of paronychia can be treated at home by applying warm, wet compresses or soaking feet in warm salty water several times a day, and using antiseptic creams or sprays. Sometimes, however, it requires antibiotics or drainage of the pus, so it's important to see your doctor if it isn't getting better, particularly if the pus isn't draining, the redness is tracking up your toe, or you feel unwell with it.

Slower growing and longer-term paronychia infections are often caused by fungi, so they're an extension of athlete's foot problems. The treatment is foot hygiene, antifungal creams and possibly tablets if these aren't helping. You can help to prevent paronychia occurring by keeping your feet as clean and dry as possible, wearing the right size running shoes and treating any athlete's foot early. If your paronychia is caused by ingrown nails, it's important to learn how best to trim your nails.

Did you know?

Paronychia is three times more common in women than it is in men. This may be due to its link with artificial nails, manicures and pedicures.

Preventing ingrown toenails

TRY THIS AT HOME

Looking after your feet is important if you want to run many miles comfortably. A toenail which grows into the soft skin around it rather than growing straight upwards can be very uncomfortable. It can also make the area more likely to get infected. Toenails do need trimming, but it's important to do it correctly. Here are some simple tips to stop nails growing into the toe:

- Don't cut your toenails too short.
- Cut the nail straight across rather than curving it round at the side of the nail.
- Make sure your running shoes have a wide enough toe box for your feet (some women may need a men's shoe to allow this).
- Don't wear socks that are too tight.
- See your GP if ingrown nails are a recurrent problem for you. Surgical options, including removing the edge of the nail, are available.

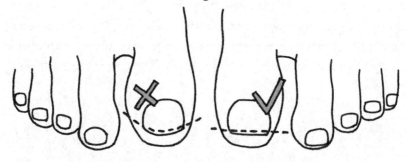

How to Cut your Toenails

LONG-TERM SKIN CONDITIONS

Q Will running get rid of my cellulite?

A There is no guarantee that any type of exercise will help reduce cellulite. Cellulite is the term used for the fatty deposits of skin around the hips and thighs. It's often lumpy in texture because of the way the underlying connective tissue, the scaffolding of skin, is stretched and pulled by the fat. Whether or not you have cellulite is largely determined by your genetics rather than your weight. Skinny people get cellulite too. Don't be fooled by expensive creams, massages and procedures promising to get rid of cellulite. They may temporarily improve skin appearance, but the best bet in the long term is to eat a healthy diet, maintain a normal body weight, and do both cardio and strength training exercise to lower body fat levels and tone the muscles underlying the fat. Many of us have cellulite. We may not like it, but it's normal and nothing to be ashamed of.

Q I have adult acne. I don't want to stop running, but I'm worried that all the sweating is making it worse.

A Sebaceous glands make sebum to keep skin and hair moist and supple. Acne occurs when the glands over-produce and the hair follicles become blocked with sebum and dead skin cells. A black-head or pustule is the result. The bacteria that naturally live on our skin then have the opportunity to infect the blocked follicles. The face is the area most likely to be affected, but the chest and back can be problematic too. Sweating heavily while running may potentially make your acne worse, because it makes the pores more likely to clog, but there are some steps you can take to minimise this risk. Always remove any make-up before you run. It's best to use a mild face wash to do this rather than just wipe it over with make-up remover. Spots often form where the skin is covered up, so tie your hair back and avoid headbands on your forehead if you're getting spots underneath them. Running packs and vest or bra straps can obstruct the skin too, but it's not so easy to avoid these. Keep your body and skin as cool as possible to minimise sweating. When you get back from your run, shower and wash your face and body thoroughly, as soon as you can, using a mild anti-bacterial wash. Always use a clean towel to dry yourself to prevent spreading bacteria. It can be a fine balance, but hopefully the benefits of running for you will outweigh any skin flare-ups. Chat to your pharmacist about which products might be best for your acne and if they aren't helping then see your GP. We often underestimate the effect that acne can have on those who suffer from it.

Real-life runners

I've had flare-ups of severe acne and rosacea, and running helped to take my mind off it. When I was running I didn't care what my skin looked like, I just enjoyed the run.

Sarah Wood, runner, writer and mum

Q Running seems to make my eczema worse. Do you have any tips for helping me to look after my skin?

A Running can both help and hinder eczema. There are lots of different types of eczema, but generally we're talking about atopic eczema, an inflammatory skin condition that usually starts in childhood. Skin gets dry, cracked, red and may weep. It's usually very itchy and can sometimes get sore and infected. If eczema flare-ups are linked to stress then you may find that running improves your skin by helping you relax. However, running can also aggravate eczema, because outdoor exercise exposes you to the elements, and wind and sun can dry out skin, making eczema worse. On top of this, skin can be irritated by sweat and further aggravated by any clothes that rub.

The key is to moisturise as frequently as you can, with a moisturiser (emollient) designed for eczema, at least three times a day. A layer of emollient before you run will help to stop skin drying out, and act as protection from sweat and chafing clothes. Shower after your run using a soap substitute, which won't dry out your skin so much, and then reapply the emollient. Experiment with which fabrics keep you coolest and rub the least – seam free clothes are good. Use a non-biological washing powder to wash your kit and consider using an extra-rinse cycle if your clothes still seem to be irritating you. There are lots of treatments available for eczema so don't suffer in silence. It's best to treat flare-ups early so seek help. It can be hard work to keep on top of eczema. Sometimes you need a trial-and-error approach, but in my experience it's very rare for eczema to prevent people running.

Did you know?

Your face turns red when you run because your body is trying to cool itself down. By dilating (expanding) the blood vessels in the skin, more blood can flow near the surface and lose its heat to the surrounding cooler air. Red faces during exercise are more common in women and more obvious in fair skinned people.

Q I have a very red face. I thought it was just from being out in all weathers but someone said I might have rosacea. Could running have caused it?

A Rosacea is a very common skin condition, but we still don't fully understand it. It affects the face and is characterised by a redness of the skin. This can come and go, but it can also stay for long periods of time or even become permanent. There may be spots, dry skin, skin thickening and broken blood vessels. It usually affects people between the ages of 40 and 60, and it can be pretty miserable for those who have it because of the way it can look. There's no cure and there are many theories as to what the cause is, including genetics, abnormalities of the blood vessels and a reaction to skin mites. Hope is not lost, though, because there do seem to be certain things which set it off, including some which are particularly relevant to runners. Strenuous exercise, strong winds, and hot and cold weather, for example, can all potentially activate rosacea, as can sun exposure and hot baths. Others on the list are stress, spicy foods, alcohol, caffeine and dairy products. If you suffer from rosacea, over time you'll probably work out what your triggers are and can avoid them where possible. Runners can shade their face from the sun with a cap or visor and wear sunscreen. In cold or windy weather a light scarf and hat might be useful. Avoiding perfumed products and looking for dietary causes can be beneficial too.

Treatment focuses on avoiding triggers, using creams to minimise redness and tablet antibiotics to reduce inflammation. If these don't help, then referral to a dermatologist is needed to explore other treatment options.

Did you know?

Sweat doesn't actually smell. It's effectively 99 per cent water with a bit of salt. The odour develops when the bacteria that live on your skin start to break the sweat down.

Q I seem to sweat much more than other runners I know. Why is this and what can I do about it?

A It's estimated that while running an endurance event in the heat, you can lose up to 10 litres of sweat in a day. How much we sweat depends on how many sweat glands we have in our skin. The average is thought to be around 3 million, but it could be as many as 5 million! The number is largely determined by our genetics – we're all made differently. There are two types of sweat gland: eccrine and apocrine. Eccrine glands are found in the dermis of the skin (see page 173) and empty their watery, salty sweat onto the skin surface. Apocrine glands are associated with hair follicles and discharge their thicker, oilier sweat into the hair follicles once puberty has commenced. This is the type of sweat you'll find in hairy areas such as your armpits or groin and this produces body odour when it meets skin bacteria.

Sweating is one of the body's ways of controlling our temperature. Heat is lost when sweat evaporates from the skin surface. It's not something we can influence, because it's controlled by the central nervous system. When you run, your body temperature increases significantly and sweating is an essential mechanism for lowering it. As you get fitter, you may find you sweat more, as your body is simply getting more efficient at thermoregulation. So potentially you could be proud of your sweating! But understandably it can be inconvenient and even embarrassing. Appropriate sportswear and good hygiene with frequent washing are obviously important. You may have tried a range of antiperspirants, but do have a chat with your pharmacist, because there are some more heavy duty ones available over the counter.

Excessive sweating when your body isn't overheating is called hyperhidrosis. This can happen all over the body or just in certain areas, such as the armpits or palms of the hands. Treatments include antiperspirants, medications, botox injections and even surgery to remove sweat glands.

TOP TIPS FOR A HEALTHY RUNNER'S SKIN

- Shower soon after running.
- Don't leave skin damp. Dry thoroughly, especially between the toes.
- Use a barrier cream to protect sore skin or problem areas while running.
- Experiment with fabrics to find which suits you best.
- Wash running kit, including socks, after one use.
- Consider alternating between two pairs of running shoes.
- Use a sunscreen with an SPF of at least 15 to protect skin from UV rays.
- Check moles regularly and report changes or new skin lesions to your GP.
- Eat a diet that includes a variety of fruit and vegetables to provide the nutrients needed for healthy skin. Top foods include avocados, nuts, seeds and fish.
- Drink plenty of water daily.

FURTHER HELP AND ADVICE

Cancer Research UK: www.cancerresearchuk.org
Melanoma UK: www.melanomauk.org.uk
British Skin Foundation: www.britishskinfoundation.org.uk
National Eczema Society: www.eczema.org
Allergy UK: www.allergyuk.org
DermNet NZ: www.dermnetnz.org
Hyperhidrosis UK: www.hyperhidrosisuk.org

CHAPTER 9

....

SELF-CARE

Being a runner and keeping well is often a fine balancing act. While we know that running makes us healthy, it can sometimes directly cause injury and illness. Trial and error, along with understanding our own bodies and a good dollop of luck, are all important in helping find the right balance for us. This chapter explores the things in everyday life that can make a difference and ensure we run well.

Our bodies aim for homeostasis, where everything is running smoothly, in equilibrium and perfect balance. So your body is continually monitoring what is going on and using multiple mechanisms to make both small and large adjustments to maintain the steady environment of homeostasis. From our thermoregulatory system, which aims to keep our core temperature constant, to our hormonal systems influencing our energy and metabolism, we are one finely tuned machine! These processes are happening day in, day out, without us being aware of them.

Sometimes the equilibrium is upset and the balance is disturbed. Both illness and injury can do this, and the body has to trigger systems to heal and repair as fast as possible. Our immune systems are incredibly complex, but very clever and effective. We're set up to succeed, with numerous ways to keep germs out. There are tiny hairs lining our airways and mucous from specialised cells, both of which trap air-borne germs. Our stomach is full of acid to kill ingested germs before they can harm us and even our skin acts as a barrier to disease. If an infection does get through, then there's an immediate response by our white blood cells, which spring into action and increase in number. White blood cells (there are several types, including neutrophils, eosinophils, basophils, monocytes and lymphocytes) can neutralise the toxins that germs produce, swallow and digest germs, or make antibodies to the germ that protect us the next time we come across it. The whole body becomes involved in clearing infections. Heart rate increases to pump blood around the body and bring cells to the areas where they're needed, and body temperature may rise to make the environment a hostile one where germs can't reproduce. The body tries to return itself to equilibrium as quickly as possible.

Our body needs energy to function. As a runner, finding the correct energy balance can be tricky. Eating the right amount of food to fuel our running and maintain our weight can be difficult for some. Getting the balance between sleep, recovery and running is also a challenge. It's very much a moving target, with our activity levels and daily lives often varying hugely from day to day. Sometimes we need to look at the bigger picture and try to find balance over a week or a month, rather than over every day. Our bodies will appreciate it if we can do this, so let's look at some of the common things upsetting our equilibrium and find out how to look after ourselves.

RUNNING AND ILLNESS

Q Should I run when I'm ill? I really don't want to get behind on my training plan.

A Not knowing whether you're well enough to run or whether you'd better give it a miss is all too familiar to a runner. The answer really depends on how unwell you are and what is wrong with you. You might have heard the saying, 'Above the neck, what the heck. In the chest, best to rest.' This is a good basic guide, but it does have its flaws and is far from comprehensive. With a mild, viral head cold, the likelihood is that a run won't hurt. It may even make you feel a little better as it can help clear nasal congestion, albeit temporarily, and it can lift your mood too. A deep sinus infection, on the other hand, even though it's above the neck, can leave you weak, dizzy and incapable of running. It's best to just be sensible – although that's often easier said than done. Here are some situations in which you should definitely miss a run:

- You have a high temperature, shivers or aches.
- You're breathless or shaky when walking.
- You feel dizzy or light-headed.
- Your resting pulse rate is higher than usual.
- You aren't properly hydrated.
- You haven't eaten a normal, full meal.
- You have a chesty cough or wheeze.
- You feel exhausted.

When you're unwell, your immune system is working hard to fight infection. It's already having its own work-out and doesn't need the extra stress that a run exerts. With illness, fevers or dehydration, your heart rate is often raised above the normal. Elevating it further with high intensity exercise can make you feel weak, dizzy or even push your heart into a potentially harmful abnormal rhythm. It's usually best to simply rest for an extra day. The fitness gains from heading out will be negligible and might even make it take longer for you to get better. Try and think of the bigger picture. Opt for light exercise or a rest day instead. If you do go out when you aren't on top form, then always take it easy and see how you feel.

Q How do I get back to running after an illness?

A It's tempting to start running as soon as you can, but it's always best to do it slowly. The last thing you want is to get ill again or injure yourself because your muscles are weak or you're still wobbly. The first thing to ask yourself is am I really better? If you're having the odd high temperature, aren't eating normally or are still coughing up green phlegm, then although you may have improved, you're still not ready to run. The longer you're unwell and the more unwell you've been, the longer it will take to get back in your trainers. If you've just had a short cold, you can probably slot back into your training within a day or two. A proper flu can put you out for three or four weeks. If you're still shattered, then just wait an extra day. Don't try to pick up where you left off. Heading out for a long run or tough interval session isn't the right thing to do. Make sure you're well fuelled and hydrated before you set off and take a bottle of water with you. It's a good idea to take your phone in case you've overestimated your health and need to bail out with a lift home. Start with a brisk walk to get properly warmed up and then break into a gentle run. Despite being desperate to crank up the pace and miles to recover lost fitness, the key is to see how you feel and not get carried away. Don't aim for a set time or distance, just have an easy run. If you're not feeling good, call it a day, head home and try again in a couple of days. Take a day of recovery after your first run, get an early night and fill up on healthy foods too. Then just build up gradually to bring you back to your pre-illness goals and you'll soon be right back on track. You'll be amazed at how quickly your fitness returns.

Q Why do I always catch a cold when I'm training for a race?

A In general, exercise boosts your immune system and helps to keep you healthy. Active people have fewer days off work than their more sedentary colleagues. However, when you've had a particularly intense session, whether that's going significantly further in your long run (usually over 90 minutes) or really pushing your body in a strenuous interval session, then there's evidence that your immune system reduces. This suppression doesn't last for long, only around 24 hours, but it may be sufficient to weaken your defences enough for a germ to take advantage of you. It's usually upper respiratory tract infections that runners catch in this situation. It's hard to avoid these, but if you're someone who is repeatedly having this problem, then it might be worth looking at your training plan. If you do your long run on a Sunday and then get up close and personal on a packed tube train every Monday morning, then it might help to move your long run to the Saturday to give your immune system an extra 24 hours to recover.

If you have children, then it's harder to resolve. Teach them to cover their coughs and sneezes with a tissue, throw it in the bin and wash their hands. Hand washing can help reduce the likelihood of catching a cold by 20 per cent, so keep washing yours too.

It's worth chatting to your pharmacist about nasal sprays that you can use at the first sign of a cold. These can help to prevent it developing. Other factors can suppress your immune system too, such as not getting enough sleep and being under stress. It's always wise to factor in an extra half an hour's sleep a night when you're training hard for an event. This will give your immune system the best chance of restoring itself, alongside helping muscle and joint repair. It's hard to relieve stress, but taking time out to relax and delegating what you can in the lead up to a race might help keep your immune system on top form. Not eating properly can have a negative effect too (see page 217).

Real-life runners

As I get older I have to take greater care of my immune system, with more rest and good food. Where once I could have kept going, fitting in mileage and intensity of training with the rest of my daily life, I now make a concerted effort to ensure I manage all the work, home and training pressures I place on my body.

Ann Butler, mum of a family of runners, and proud member of Ramsbottom Running Club

Q How do I know if I'm overtraining?

A It's normal to feel tired when you're training hard, especially if you're combining it with a busy work and home life. But if you find that you plateau in your running, become unable to match or improve your times, or lack the endurance for distance, then it might be time to take a step back. Is there a mismatch between what you are demanding of your body and the recovery time you are giving it? It can be a fine balance. It's usually enough to reassess your plan and perhaps take a short period of rest, or cut back on your intensity and frequency of running if you think you're overdoing things.

Sometimes, excess training can be more serious and begin to affect your body in a more harmful way. You may have heard of Over Training Syndrome (OTS). This is the term used for a condition involving prolonged overtraining. It's rare and usually seen in professional athletes. It can be career-ending for some of them, as excessive training demands, coupled with the inability of the body to recover adequately from exercise during rest, can lead to problems in multiple body systems. Physiological, immunological, hormonal and psychological systems can all be affected, and also all play a role in recovery. While true OTS is rare, it's important to know what the symptoms of excessive training on the body can be, in case you begin to identify them in yourself. Having one or more of these symptoms doesn't mean you have OTS, but you would be well advised to assess your running and recovery balance, and consider seeing your GP to discuss whether you need any blood tests to rule out underlying medical conditions:

- Constantly feeling tired.
- Underperforming despite resting.
- Frequently getting ill.
- Frequently getting injured.
- Not being able to sleep despite being tired.
- Finding it hard to concentrate.
- Feeling low or irritable in mood.
- Lacking motivation.
- Not feeling refreshed by recovery.

Running safely with a medical condition

TRY THIS AT HOME

If you have a long-term medical condition and are a runner, then it's a good idea to be as prepared as you can be, to minimise any risks that running might pose. Here are some simple tips you can follow to help you exercise more safely:

continued overleaf ▶

- Fill in your details on the back of your race bib. Marshals, other runners and paramedics will look here for information about medical conditions and emergency contacts.
- Register with a medical alert provider, carry a card and wear a medical alert tag or piece of jewellery. This will quickly give important information about your condition to care-givers. Some services provide 24-hour telephone back up giving more detailed health information to health care professionals and include a translation service, which is useful if you're racing abroad.
- If you have a condition that may affect you on your run, such as diabetes or epilepsy, then inform your run buddy or running club leader as to what might happen and what they need to do if you are in difficulty.
- Always carry your mobile phone with you – you never know when you might need to call for help. There are apps that allow friends and family to find your location, and even those that will send an alert to someone you nominate if you have been still for a certain period of time or you activate the call for help function. If you're running alone, tell someone where you're going and when you plan to get back.
- Remember to carry any medication that you might need during your run. Inhalers for asthma or glucose tablets for low blood sugars can usually fit into running kit pockets. Take your everyday medications regularly, as prescribed.
- Be aware that a change in dose of medication can sometimes affect the control of your medical condition. For example, a higher dose of blood pressure tablet can initially make you feel dizzy. Check with your doctor whether there are any likely side-effects and how these may affect your running. It may simply be a case of leaving a few days for things to settle before you run and then taking it slowly.
- Be prepared to be flexible and adapt your running plans to account for your medical condition. Cut back if you don't feel on top form and see your nurse or doctor if you are unsure about any symptoms or side-effects.

Q Will running reduce my risk of cancer?

While there's no guarantee that if you run regularly you won't get cancer, it's important to know that it can reduce your risk of many types of cancer. To gain health benefits it's recommended that people do at least 150 minutes per week of moderate intensity exercise – that's exercise that makes you feel a bit out of breath. Running is classed as vigorous intensity exercise and the target for that is 75 minutes, which most runners fulfil easily in an average week. There may be increased benefits for exceeding that target for some cancers, but there are no clear guidelines yet. The type of risk reductions you can expect from running regularly throughout your life (not just a one-off 5km run) include: breast cancer – 20 to 30 per cent; colorectal cancer – 20 per cent; and bladder cancer – 20 per cent. Exercise is a powerful medicine. While we can't change our genetics and other factors which determine our cancer risk, we can alter our lifestyles, and running fits the bill perfectly for an accessible and effective form of exercise. Exercise can also reduce the risk of certain cancers returning after treatment has been completed.

Did you know?

Exercise helps people with cancer tolerate the side-effects of cancer treatment, including fatigue, nausea and low mood. If they aren't feeling up to running, then even a short walk can give benefits, so why not ask your friend with cancer if they fancy a stroll rather than a coffee?

RUNNING AND INJURIES

Q How long should you have off running when you have an injury?

A The body has an amazing ability to repair itself. Everyone will heal at their own rate and recovery times vary from person to person. They also depend on which body tissues have been injured and how severely. The most frequent everyday injuries in runners are those that include muscles and ligaments. Pulled and torn muscles are called strains and overstretched ligaments are called sprains. As a very rough guide, you can expect to be off running for a week with a mild muscle strain and a month for a more severe one. Sprains take longer, so expect a month for a mild sprain and three to four months for a severe one. It's incredibly frustrating to be injured and tempting to just carry on and run as soon as you can, but it's vital to respect injuries and allow the body time to repair and strengthen the injured area. This will minimise the risk of re-injury.

When the acute pain has eased, start gently stretching and moving the injured area. If you've had a sprain, particularly a severe one, then you would benefit from seeing a physiotherapist to give you specific exercises to help strengthen the area and guide you back to running.

You shouldn't even consider running until you are pain free and can walk normally without discomfort. When you do restart then build up very gradually and be guided by how the injury feels. Any aching, twinges or increased swelling suggests you might need to cut back a bit or rest for a while longer. Patience is key!

Using PRICE

Serious injuries where you're unable to weight-bear, clearly have a broken bone or are in a lot of pain obviously need urgent medical assessment. Sometimes, however, you aren't too sure of the severity or you're confident that it's a more minor injury and you want to treat it yourself. In this situation, follow PRICE for strains and sprains to reduce pain and help healing:

Protect Prevent any further injury to the area. Don't try to carry on running. Phone for a lift or get assistance from a fellow runner.

Rest Don't use the injured area. Use pain as your guide. If it's hurting then don't do it!

Ice Apply cold packs or ice to the area. Don't put ice directly against the skin. Always wrap it in fabric such as a tea towel to prevent skin damage. Apply it for 15 minutes every two hours. Avoid applying heat to the area for 72 hours.

Compress Gently squeeze the injured area with a bandage. You can buy tubular elasticated bandages from the pharmacy. They'll advise you as to which size and compression strength you need. Take them off at night. Don't massage the area in the first 72 hours as it may increase the swelling.

Elevate Injured tissues swell as fluid accumulates and this can cause pain. Let gravity help you and keep the injured area raised. This may mean putting your ankle up on a chair so it's higher than your hip or wearing a sling for an injured wrist.

Use PRICE for three days, but if you aren't getting relief, the pain and swelling is increasing and you suspect more than just a sprain or strain, then get a medical opinion.

Q What painkillers are best for runners?

A When rest and ice aren't giving you enough relief then you can reduce pain with an analgesic (painkilling medication). The safest one to use is paracetamol. Most people don't realise that paracetamol has some anti-inflammatory actions as well as directly reducing pain. The dose for adults over 50 kilograms is 1 gram (two of the 500 milligram tablets) up to four times a day. You should leave a minimum of four to six hours between doses and not take more than 4 grams (eight tablets) in 24 hours. There aren't many medical situations where paracetamol is not advised, but they include liver damage from alcoholism, long-term liver disease and interactions with some epilepsy and cancer medications. It's safe to take paracetamol on an empty stomach, making it a good choice for injuries during running when you may not have eaten for several hours.

The other common analgesics that you can buy over the counter are Non-Steroidal Anti-Inflammatories (NSAIDs). The most frequently used is ibuprofen. NSAIDs mainly work by reducing inflammation, which is an effective way to reduce pain from inflamed and swollen tissues. However, there is now an opinion that using NSAIDs within 48 hours of an injury might slow down the healing process. The thinking is that the body intentionally activates inflammation to draw cells and fluids to the area to promote healing. Disrupting and preventing this may slow recovery. So paracetamol seems the best option in those first few days.

There are also quite a few cautions that need to be considered with NSAIDs. Check with your pharmacist or doctor whether you can use them if you have ever had stomach ulcers, allergy to aspirin, asthma (they can provoke an attack in some people), heart disease, kidney disease, inflammatory bowel disease, are breast feeding or are taking any medications that thin your blood, such as warfarin. You should not use ibuprofen if you are pregnant. The usual recommended dose is 200 to 400 milligrams three times a day.

It's best to avoid taking it on an empty stomach. Anti-inflammatories can also be given locally, through a cream or gel which is rubbed into the skin. This doesn't reduce the risk of all side-effects or cautions, because the active ingredient is still absorbed into the bloodstream (see page 69).

Did you know?

Swelling after an injury isn't all bad news. In the first 48 hours the body intentionally causes inflammation in the damaged area. The extra tissue fluids immobilise the joint and restrict its movement, which allows healing and protects it from further injury. The fluids are also packed with cells brought into the area to stop further bleeding from torn blood vessels, to remove waste products and debris, and to stimulate growth and regeneration.

Q Why do I keep getting injured?

A Are you one of those unlucky people who seems to move from one injury to another, doesn't ever get a long stretch of training and has DNS (Did Not Start) recorded on multiple races? Is it all down to luck? Why do some people get injured all the time and others never seem to? There are multiple things to consider when it comes to recurrent injuries. Genetics and susceptibility to injury is one of them. We can't change the genetic code that determines the exact make-up of our bones, tendons, cartilage and muscles. There are professional sports teams who do use genetic information to tailor individual training programmes, so who knows, in the future there may be similar options for recreational runners. In the meantime, and more importantly, there are many factors that we can change and influence to reduce the risk of recurrent injury. Here are some reasons why you might be repeatedly getting injured. It's easy to see how you can correct each one:

- **Returning too soon after injury** Repair may take longer than you think and even when a muscle is pain free and functioning normally, it is still healing. Rushing back and picking up where you left off leaves you vulnerable to further injury. Be patient and take rehabilitation seriously.

- **One thing leads to another** Having an injury alters the way you run, walk and generally hold yourself. This can put strain on other parts of your body, making them injury prone. For example, a knee injury might result in a foot or hip injury on the other side of the body. Get significant injuries diagnosed and allow adequate recovery time.

- **Ignoring niggles** It's tempting to just keep running. After all, you can't stop with every little twinge. However, if you're someone who always turns a blind eye to low-grade pain and aches then it's sensible to listen to your body, take two or three days off and then return with a lower running intensity and distance to see if they persist. Get assessed if they do.

- **Underlying weakness** It might be that you have weaknesses in your body that aren't apparent in everyday life, but when the extra load of running is added they become significant. This can result in poor running technique. Weak glute muscles from a sedentary lifestyle, for example, leave you at increased risk of multiple injuries, including Iliotibial Band Syndrome (see page 167). A physiotherapist assessment will pick up any weaknesses and can direct strength training.

- **Inadequate warm-ups** The jury is out on how much warming up influences injury risk, but if you're someone who gets multiple injuries and skimps on warm-ups then it's definitely worth changing your routine to see if it helps.

- **No variation in training** An interesting 2016 study of marathon runners found that regular interval training may reduce the risk of injury. Consider varying your training plan to include intervals as well as strength work and cross training.

- **Lack of recovery time** Not allowing your body sufficient time to recover from training or increasing the load too rapidly could leave it susceptible to injury. Recovery time increases with age, so consider adding an extra rest day into your week and always increase training loads gradually.
- **Lifestyle issues** Sometimes it's not the running, it's everything else! Are you getting enough sleep? Are you stressed? Is your diet poor? All of these factors have a role to play in how your body copes with a training load. If you're stressed, sleep deprived and eating junk food, it's going to be hard for adequate recovery and repair to take place. Always look at the bigger picture.

Real-life runners

There were times when I would despair with the injuries. It seemed unfair when I was trying to improve my health and wellbeing yet was just ending up crocked! I also know that I should have listened to my own body and not been driven by my own obsession to absolutely always complete the distance my plan said. I fundamentally compromised my Dublin Marathon 2020 by pushing my last 20-mile long run when I should have stopped. I did finish the marathon, but tapering for it was basically no running and investing in massage, a chiropractor and anti-inflammatory gel!

Mike Whelan, runner and Leinster Rugby fanatic

Q How quickly will I lose my fitness when I'm off running?

A It's so frustrating to be injured or ill and you can almost feel your fitness draining out of you with every day that passes. Studies on this topic, which is called detraining or deconditioning, are pretty mixed and each person will have an individual response to time away from running. The good news, however, is that if you are a regular runner, although your aerobic fitness initially drops quite quickly, after a few days of inactivity it levels off and doesn't just keep going down and down. It won't fall back to that of an inactive person, which gives you a higher baseline fitness. You'll lose fitness more slowly than a more inactive person too. There's also the bonus that you will bounce back to fitness more quickly. It's worth also considering your structural fitness, meaning your muscle strength. This declines more slowly than your aerobic fitness, but to prevent injury it's important to build it back up prior to returning to running.

Some encouraging news for those that are currently side-lined is to know that you can maintain the majority of your fitness with as little as one high intensity work-out a week. This is a good reason to do whatever exercise you can. For example, if running is out then a swim or some time on the static bike will benefit you. Don't forget you can do some form of core work or strength exercises while injured to maintain your structural fitness. In summary, with a good baseline fitness and a consistent training habit, a week off due to illness or injury isn't going to be much of a problem. More extended time away can be counteracted by keeping up some form of maintenance activity and knowing that you will return to fitness pretty quickly when you are ready to.

Q How many rest days do I need each week?

This is often a case of trial and error. While some people can get away with a running streak of a year or more, there are those who need frequent days of rest. There are a few factors to consider, your running experience being one of them. Beginners who set off with great enthusiasm and run numerous times a week can quickly become injured, whereas a seasoned runner could easily cope with the same frequency. Recovery days in those early stages, while the body adapts to running, are essential. Adaptation and repair takes place when you rest. An overnight sleep may be enough for some bodies to go through this process, but others require longer. Our repair processes slow down as we age and it's not uncommon for older runners to feel they need more recovery days than when they were younger.

Obviously, how much you push yourself will affect your need for recovery too. A gentle 5km won't need as much recovery time as running a marathon PB. It's best to take an overview of your training. If you're remaining well, enjoying your running and making any gains that you want, then your recovery is probably adequate. If you're new to running, finding runs harder than you feel you should, or are really cranking up the frequency or intensity of your running, then it's advisable to factor in at least one or two rest days a week. Recovery is an important part of training so should not be associated with guilt.

Did you know?

Between 37 per cent and 56 per cent of recreational runners who train regularly and run the odd long-distance race will get injured each year.

RUNNING AND FOOD

Q What's the best diet for a runner?

A There are emerging, widespread and well-advertised benefits to certain diets. Some runners following vegan and LCHF (Low Carbohydrate High Fat) diets report increased endurance capacity, quicker recovery times and easier weight maintenance. The research is growing, but can be contradictory. It is a very confusing time for the general public when it comes to diet and nutrition, with much conflicting advice. I don't feel this book should tell you what you should be eating. It's a very personal thing. As a runner, the best diet is the one that works for you; one that gives you enough energy to fuel your runs, that allows you to improve as a runner (if that is your goal) and supplies the nutrients your body needs to repair itself; one that keeps you healthy, that's practical and affordable for you and that sits comfortably with your own environmental conscience. It should give you pleasure too. If you're ticking all those boxes, then that's perfect. If not, then it's up to you to look at alternatives and make adjustments. It's just important to know that you can't put rubbish in and expect excellence out. If your diet is poor, for whatever reason, then there is lots of unleashed potential that you could gain from, both in terms of your running and your general health, so be pro-active, and explore your options and what might work for you.

Q Why doesn't running help me lose weight?

A Many people start running thinking that it will be a good way to lose weight and the majority are disappointed. While for some running can result in shedding pounds, for others it actually results in weight gain, which can be incredibly frustrating and disappointing. The first and most important point is that if you have increased your fitness through running and become more active than you were, then you have improved your health, regardless of what the scales say. Yes, some of the benefits of exercise come from losing weight, but many of them are completely independent. Using weight loss as a marker of your fitness gains is not a good idea. By increasing your activity levels you will have boosted your muscle mass (which may be responsible for some of your weight gain). This results in an increased number of myokines, which are released from muscle during exercise and have an anti-inflammatory effect in the body, reducing the risk of many serious medical conditions, such as type 2 diabetes and cancer. By exercising more you will have also reduced your visceral fat. This is the harmful fat around your internal organs and it causes inflammation in the body. It is responsive to physical activity and by lowering the amount of it you will again have reduced internal inflammation and improved your health.

So running can build muscle, which may make the scales read higher, and it can also make you really hungry. It's so easy for the overwhelming hunger that strikes after a run (also known as runger) to result in larger portions, extra carbohydrates and multiple snacks. The cravings are real! It's also easy to overestimate how much you've burned off during a run (approximately 100 calories per mile) and even easier to overcompensate with food. The same can be said for activity levels. Knowing that you have been for a run can lower the amount of exercise you do during the rest of the day – you may feel you've earned the right to lie on the sofa for the rest of the day. This may be a subconscious behaviour, but it still leads to using fewer calories and weight gain. Don't forget that if you're using sports gels or drinks they will contain additional calories that are easily forgotten. In fact, you may return from a run without a calorie deficit at all. It's common to see some weight loss initially, but then it may plateau and even increase over time. This can be a result of the body adapting and becoming more efficient at using fuel, resulting in a slower metabolism. Throwing in some high intensity work and building muscle can help to counteract this. The moral of the story, though, is to be wary of what the scales tell you. Judge your fitness and body by how you feel and look, and find your own balance between running and eating.

Q I run every day and train hard but my running isn't going very well at the moment. I eat really healthily because I don't want to become overweight but I'm conscious I might not be eating enough for all the exercise I do.

A Whatever your size, if there is a mismatch between the energy you are putting into your body and the energy you are expending, then this can potentially cause problems. There is a fine balance needed to remain healthy. You may have heard of the term RED-S, which stands for Relative Energy Deficiency in Sport. This is used to describe a situation where disordered eating results in a negative energy balance and subsequent health consequences. Disordered eating includes specific eating disorders such as anorexia and bulimia, but also includes any poor relationship with food leading to eating habits that don't provide the body with enough energy for training and for basic bodily functions. Clearly, low energy availability will impact running performance, but RED-S is more serious than that. The body starts shutting down some of its normal functions to conserve energy. Many systems will be affected. The most significant for women is the fall in oestrogen levels, resulting in amenorrhea (a lack of menstrual periods) and osteoporosis (low bone mass). Amenorrhoea (see page 121) can lead to fertility problems. Osteoporosis leaves people susceptible to bone fracture and collapse. The combination of an eating disorder, osteoporosis and amenorrhoea used to be called the 'female athlete triad', but we now use the term RED-S because we realise that any type of disordered eating is significant. The consequences are much more widespread than just bones and periods, and men can be affected too. People with RED-S often underperform and are at high risk of injuries. There can be disruption of digestion, mood, the immune system and also negative effects on the cardiovascular system.

If you are struggling with balancing eating and training and think you may have RED-S, then it's important that you seek help. Specialist input and advice is needed to diagnose and treat RED-S. Your next step should be to make an appointment with your GP who can refer you to a specialist clinic if required.

Did you know?

You can't tell if someone has an eating disorder by looking at them. People who are underweight, overweight or of normal weight can all be affected. Never judge.

RUNNING AND DAILY LIFE

Q I love running, but I'm generally just so tired all the time and don't have enough energy for it. Should I go to the doctor?

A Feeling tired all the time is one of the most common reasons people see their GP. It's most definitely a sign of the times, with huge pressures and expectations being put on us from both society and ourselves. While there are medical conditions that cause fatigue, the diagnosis more often than not comes down to lifestyle. Being anaemic (having low numbers of red blood cells) and hypothyroidism (an underactive thyroid) are the two most common medical causes of fatigue, particularly in women. These can be diagnosed by a blood test so if you suspect that your fatigue may be down to more than just a hectic life or you have any of the following symptoms, then you should see your GP:

- You're passing more urine than normal or are constantly thirsty.
- You're losing or gaining weight without a change in your diet.
- You have night sweats (and aren't menopausal).
- You have any lumps in your armpits, groin or neck.
- You've had a change in your normal bowel habit or blood in your stools.
- You're more out of breath than usual.
- You've been getting palpitations, dizzy spells or chest pains.
- You have heavy periods.
- You're excessively tired every day and aren't able to function normally.

If there's no underlying medical condition then it's helpful to know that even if you don't feel you have the energy for a run, it might be just the thing you need. Yes, sometimes a rest is best, but running can give you an energy boost. It may be that some time away from life, either solo or with running friends, will refresh you and give you a feeling of wellbeing. It's also important to do what you can to ensure you're sleeping as well as possible and eating high-quality foods in enough quantity to fuel your daily life and running. Stress is exhausting too. It may not be one overwhelming issue, just a long-term, low-level stress that is sapping your energy (see page 5). Trying to get the right balance in life isn't always easy, but it's essential to prioritise yourself sometimes.

Q I know that running is supposed to help sleep. I run regularly, but I still can't sleep.

A People who exercise generally sleep better than those who don't. But, we're all different and insomnia is thought to be a problem for around one third of the UK population. It's particularly difficult if you're a shift worker or have children who can be little sleep thieves. With respect to running, if you exercise late in the day it might be worth changing the time you run. While some studies show that evening exercise doesn't affect sleep, there are certainly people who find that the surge of adrenalin produced by high intensity exercise makes it hard for them to unwind and get off to sleep. Other things that you should avoid before bed are heavy meals (allow a couple of hours for digestion), looking at a screen (have at least an hour screen-free before sleep) and caffeine (it's best not to have any after 4pm). Alcohol can also affect both the quality and quantity of your sleep.

To try and help you sleep, make sure your bedroom is dark and cool; that it's not cluttered with things that will make you think about all the things you need to do the next day; and that you've had a period of winding down doing something relaxing, such as a bath or reading. Relaxation is key – you need to quieten your thoughts. There are lots of relaxation apps you can try, including ones that play the sound of the sea or rain to act as white noise and help you drift off.

Practise sleep hygiene, which means going to bed and getting up at the same time every day to get your body into a healthy rhythm and habit. Avoid napping in the day, even if the urge is strong! If you can't sleep or you wake in the night and can't get back to sleep, then try to stay calm. Worrying about not sleeping will make it worse. Lie quietly and do some relaxation. If half an hour has passed and you're still not asleep, then get up. Don't do what so many patients over the years told me they did – make a cup of tea! You need to avoid stimulation and caffeine, so do something you dislike and find boring, such as ironing. You don't want to reward yourself. Return to bed after a while and repeat the relaxation techniques.

Sleep disturbance is common and usually short-lived. It's often related to life events, but it's worth knowing that there may be a long lag between the event and the sleep issues. Having a longer-term sleep problem is dreadful and can have a huge impact on your life. There are sometimes other health conditions underlying poor sleep. The hormonal fluctuations around the time of the menopause (see page 130) can cause restless nights for women and an over-active bladder (see page 103) can mean many night-time wakings. Mood disorders and medication side-effects may also be to blame. See your doctor if this is the case. Remember too that it's entirely normal to hardly sleep a wink before an important race!

Did you know?

Exercise is a powerful anti-ageing tool. As we get older, our telomeres (the little caps on the end of our chromosomes which protect the genetic material inside) shorten. Exercise has been shown to slow down the rate the telomeres shorten, so our DNA is protected for longer and we age more slowly.

Q I hate running when it's hot. I sweat so much and get tired really quickly. I'm running a marathon this summer. Do you have any tips?

A Some of us tolerate running in the heat better than others. You'll hear of runners heading off to the Marathon de Sables spending time running in a heat chamber to prepare their bodies. The most helpful thing is to practise so our bodies adapt, but as we don't have long, reliably hot summers in the UK this is hard to achieve. Here are some things you can try to make your summer marathon easier:

- **Adjust your plan** First up, be realistic. If the temperature is set to soar and hot running isn't your thing, then don't be over ambitious with your race goal. You will most likely have to slow down. It can be a risky business aiming for a PB in conditions that aren't optimal for you.
- **Pick the right gear** Light, breathable fabrics that you've practised in are best. Women are sometimes reluctant to run in shorts, but they're a lot cooler than capris or tights. Vest tops will let your skin breathe more, but some people prefer a t-shirt to keep the sun off their shoulders.
- **Use cream and lube** You'll need sunscreen on any exposed skin. Avoid too much on your forehead because if it runs into your eyes it can sting. Use lubricant on areas that are prone to chafing, such as inner thighs (if you're in shorts) and vest and bra strap areas. You'll be glad of it when your clothes get wet with sweat and water.
- **Hats and glasses** A cap with a brim to keep the sun off your face can be a lifesaver or use a visor if you prefer to leave the top of your head uncovered.
- **Start cool** Precooling means lowering your core body temperature before you exercise and there is evidence that it can help performance in the heat. While applying cooling packs or sitting in cold water before a race isn't practical, you can drink very cold drinks or ice slushies to cool you from the inside out.

- **Keep cool** On hot days, races will often have shower sprays that you can run through or wet sponges and ice being handed out. Put some ice in your cap, and let it melt and slowly trickle down your neck for a couple of miles. You can put ice into your drink bottle too.
- **Drink to thirst** You'll need more fluids than you would on a cool day, but don't put yourself at risk of hyponatraemia (low blood sodium levels) by over drinking (see page 70).

Q I had to pull out of a half marathon recently, because I got so hot. Someone said I probably had heat exhaustion. Is this the same as heat stroke?

A Heat exhaustion can lead to heat stroke if it isn't treated. Our body has a core temperature (around 37°C) at which all its systems can function normally. The body has numerous thermoregulation mechanisms that it employs to keep the temperature as stable as possible, such as sweating, faster breathing and dilating up blood vessels to take as much blood to the surface of the skin as possible. When you exercise, your core temperature increases. Your skin is vital to help get rid of excess heat, but if it's a particularly hot day and your skin temperature rises too, then it becomes harder to shed heat.

The first thing that might happen when your core temperature increases, but is still less than 40°C, is heat cramps. You might feel very thirsty, have a fast heart rate and your muscles will cramp, but you will otherwise be OK. Rest, cooling and rehydrating with an isotonic electrolyte drink may be all that is necessary. Next is heat exhaustion. Your core temperature is high, but still below 41°C. Your body is still trying to get rid of heat so you'll probably be hot, flushed and sweaty with a fast heart rate, and you won't feel well. Weakness, dizziness and a headache are common with heat exhaustion, but you may also feel sick, clumsy or irritable.

The next stage is heatstroke, where the core temperature is at least 40.6°C and, frighteningly, the body's mechanisms for shedding heat may have switched off. Confusion and poor co-ordination are prominent. Seizures may occur. Rather than feeling overheated you may feel cold and stop sweating (you are usually in a critical condition by this stage). Once the core temperature goes over 41.5°C then things are very serious, with many organs in the body at risk of failing, potentially leading to severe damage or even death. Heatstroke obviously needs to be urgently treated in hospital where steps will be taken to rapidly cool the person, and to monitor and support their organ function. Interestingly, although rapid cooling helps, the target temperature is 39°C, which is above normal body temperature. There's the risk of a rebound temperature if it goes too low too quickly.

The key is to avoid heat cramps and heat exhaustion. Follow the steps to running cool in the question above. Knowing how to treat heat exhaustion and prevent it progressing to heat stroke is vital, and potentially life-saving.

Treating heat exhaustion

TRY THIS AT HOME

Treating heat exhaustion can stop it progressing to the serious condition of heatstroke. Here's what to do to help someone with heat exhaustion:

1. Move them to a cool place. Find somewhere out of the sun or a car with air conditioning.
2. Lie them down and elevate their legs above the level of their heart.
3. Give them fluids to drink – water, rehydration drinks, whatever is available, and if it's cold then even better.
4. Loosen clothing to let air circulate around them.
5. Use cool water to sponge them down and fan them with whatever you have available. If you have access to cold packs, then you can put them on the soles of their feet and palms of their hands.

continued overleaf ▶

Q I'm a fair-weather runner. I hate being cold, but this year I have to run through the winter because I have a spring marathon. How can I keep warm?

A Tempting though it is to head out in a down jacket, dressed for the Arctic, you'll end up overheating. Running will make you warm, so dress for the second mile rather than the first. Check the outside temperature. It's often warmer than you think and you'll soon figure out how many layers you need for each temperature and wind chill. Base layers are really important for keeping your core temperature warm, so it's worth investing in a really good one. On the coldest days, a woollen base such as merino wool will provide warmth, but also wick away sweat and dry quickly. Layers are great. They trap air which provides insulation. You can also take layers on and off, and tie them around your waist if you need to.

Your body temperature may feel hotter and colder at different points on a long run, particularly if the weather changes or you find yourself running into the wind. Tops and jackets with long zips up the front mean you can unzip when you want to let air in to cool you down or zip up if you're feeling chilly. Windproof jackets are a good idea too. Look for thermal running tights – some have a fleecy lining. These can make a big difference if you're someone (like me) who ends up with freezing thighs and buttocks.

For the coldest days, a hat with a thermal lining is a great addition to keep you toasty – a lot of heat is lost through your head. A light scarf stops the cold air going down your neck and you can cover your nose and mouth with it too. Having freezing cold fingers can be miserable so gloves are essential, particularly for those suffering with Raynaud's disease (see page 36). Pre-warm your hat, scarf and gloves on the radiator.

Don't forget, though, as soon as you stop running, your body temperature will fall quickly. In combination with the wet sweat on you, you'll soon feel really cold. Do a cool-down run and walk to bring your body temperature gradually back to normal. Make sure you have plenty of warm layers to put on if you're away from home, and hop in a warm shower and have a hot drink as soon as you can. Don't let the winter weather put you off. It's a great time to be running. A spring running goal will keep you going out on the worst of days. You'll soon get used to it, and find out what and how much you need to wear.

Q I don't have much time to go running, so I don't usually bother warming up.

A I think lots of runners are guilty of this and either skip a warm-up completely or just go a bit more slowly for their first mile. It is worth knowing what the benefits of warming up are so you can make up your own mind as to whether it's something you want to make time for or not. While warming up won't completely get rid of those 'toxic ten minutes' that you experience at the start of a run, it will introduce your body to the idea that it's about to work hard, improve elasticity of connective tissues, elevate your heart rate and prepare the lungs for what's to come. There's a phenomenon called post activation potentiation which means that when you have asked a muscle to contract once, it will contract with a greater force the next time. So, if performance is important to you, then warming up is vital. A warm-up can be beneficial to joints too. Synovial fluid circulates in your joints to lubricate and cushion them, and this is stimulated by activity, so beginning gently and gradually building up intensity will allow time for this to happen.

Something that you may be unaware of is how warming up benefits your nervous system. Taking time to fire up the pathways between your brain and your muscles and joints can help to lower your risk of injury.

Activating muscles, sending feedback about joint position and fine-tuning co-ordination will reduce your risk of tripping and falling.

Finally, don't forget that warming up your mind is important too. Think about what you want to achieve, how far you have come and the tone you want to set for your run. You might need positive thoughts and imagery for a race, or deep breaths and thought blocking if you're running away from a busy day. Either way a bit of time to focus your mind can help you get the most out of your run.

Warm-ups don't need to be complicated and you don't have to do them before you go out or on the doorstep. Ten minutes to walk briskly and run slowly followed by some dynamic stretches is enough. You might find it's ten minutes well spent.

Did you know?

Dynamic stretches are stretches that take a joint through its whole range of movement. They include arm and leg swings, hip rotations and trunk twists.

Q I run three times a week. Is this enough to keep me healthy?

A The Chief Medical Officers' guidelines for physical activity state that 150 minutes of moderate intensity activity or 75 minutes of vigorous intensity activity is the recommended amount for good health. Running is vigorous activity so three 25-minute runs a week will tick that box. However, you shouldn't spend the rest of your week being inactive. Your three runs a week don't cancel out the need to do anything else.

The guidelines now have a new emphasis on muscle-strengthening activities, which should be done on at least two days a week. Running helps to build muscular endurance and strength, particularly in the legs. However, including a couple of specific muscle-building sessions a week will ensure that you maintain muscle and bone mass as you age. This can be done with simple exercises at home, using your own body weight to do exercises such as wall sits and press-ups. You can use resistance bands and weights too, but it's important to use a good technique so a session with an instructor to advise you is a good idea to get you started.

The other really important recommendation is to reduce your sedentary time. Too much time spent sitting is bad for your health, increasing the risks of many major diseases, such as heart disease, cancer and in particular type 2 diabetes. With prolonged sitting your body goes into storage mode, holding on to fat. This can be prevented by simply getting up and moving around for a couple of minutes every half an hour or so. Moving frequently also helps to reduce the inflammation in your body. Inflammation results from early cell death when unused energy is released as free radicals, which damage and destroy cells.

If you're over 65 years of age you should also take part in balance and co-ordination activities at least twice a week. Those neural pathways need to be activated or they shut down. Currently there's only sufficient evidence to definitely recommend this for those over 65, but I believe anyone over 40 would benefit from balance and co-ordination training. This could be a yoga or tai chi class, home exercises such as spending time standing one leg or balancing on a curb when you're out for a walk.

Being active enough for good health means taking care of all these aspects of activity and not solely relying on a quick run every few days. That is far better than nothing, though, and should be applauded, because four in 10 adults in England don't reach the 150-minute target and one quarter are classed as inactive, doing less than 30 minutes a week.

Balance and co-ordination

TRY THIS AT HOME

Balance and co-ordination abilities are quickly lost if you don't use them. Try this exercise at home. You may want to do it holding on to something initially:

- Stand up tall with your feet together, shoulders back and bottom tucked in.

continued overleaf ▶

- With your arms by your side and keeping your body still, slowly lift one leg and bend it until your foot is level with your knee.
- Hold this position for the count of 20.
- Now close your eyes. Try to remain in this position for another count of 20.
- Repeat on the other leg.
- When you've mastered this, try doing it at the same time as brushing your teeth!

TOP TIPS FOR A HEALTHY RUNNER'S BALANCE

Running, and keeping well and free of injuries, is a continuous game of balance. Here are my tips for keeping the scales even:

- Rest when you're ill or injured.
- Get injuries diagnosed if they aren't resolving quickly.
- Take your time coming back from illness or injury.
- Train progressively, but flexibly too, so you can cut back if you need to.
- Don't skimp on the warm-up.
- Do what you can to get a good night's sleep and add in extra if you're training hard.
- Dress for the weather.
- Add in muscle-strengthening work, balance and co-ordination activities and cut down your sedentary time.
- Eat a diet that works for you, and provides you with the energy and nutrients to fuel your active life.
- Be proud that you're a runner and doing amazing things for your health and wellbeing, both now and in the future.

FURTHER HELP AND ADVICE

NHS website: www.nhs.uk

Patient: www.patient.info

Netdoctor: www.netdoctor.co.uk

Macmillan Cancer Support: www.macmillan.org.uk

Sleepstation: www.sleepstation.org.uk/articles/

Beat Eating Disorders: www.beateatingdisorders.org.uk

Trainbrave: www.trainbrave.org

ACKNOWLEDGEMENTS

I really hope you have enjoyed reading *Run Well* and found some tips and advice to help you on your running journey. We all need help sometimes and I have certainly needed it in abundance writing this book! Thank you to all the wonderful runners who gave me quotes and to my running friends Sally, Jo, Tamsin, Louise, Lisa, Rochelle and Ann for being my chapter reviewers. Thanks also to Bernie and Laraine for their input on the basic life support section. Huge thanks to the amazing runners who waded through proof copies to be able to offer me endorsements, I feel honoured and really appreciate your time and seal of approval.

I'm so grateful to all the team at Bloomsbury, especially my editors Charlotte Croft and Sarah Skipper. I was so excited they published my first book, *Sorted: The Active Woman's Guide to Health* and delighted they wanted to help me realise this vision of creating a health handbook for all runners.

Thank you to all my followers on social media who motivate and spur me on every day with their passion for running and never fail to 'like' all my far from perfect running selfies! I love to chat about running so do come and say hello on my social media accounts or on my blog drjulietmcgrattan.com.

Thanks to all those people in my life who've 'got my back' with special mention to friends Tamsin, Nicky, Jennie, Lisa, Vicki and Louise. To Christina Neal, Lisa Jackson, Rhalou Allerhand, Joe Williams, Vicki Broadbent, Moire O'Sullivan and Nell McAndrew, thank you for all the support, encouragement and opportunities you have given me. And to the wonderful team at 261 Fearless, it's an honour to work with you to bring running to so many women around the world. Kathrine Switzer, Edith Zuschmann and Horst von Bohlen, thank you for teaching me so much about running, life and business, you are truly my inspirations.

An extra special thank you to my family who raised an eyebrow when I announced my next writing challenge, but then got fully behind me to help me get to the end. To Ken, Joseph, Thomas and Molly, thanks for all the love and fun, for waiting at finish lines and for being patient while I wrote. You're the best!

If you have enjoyed *Run Well*, I'd be so grateful if you would leave me a review at the place you buy your books online. I know it's adding to your to-do list but it makes so much difference to authors. Thank you so much.

And finally, a huge thank you to all of you in the running community. You always brighten my day. Enjoy the wonderful gift of running everybody and make sure you run well!

REFERENCES

Chapter 1: The Head

Berk, M. Williams, L.J. Jacka, F.N. O'Neil, A. Pasco, J. Moylan, S. Allen, N.B. Stuart, A.L. Hayley, A.C. Byrne, M.L. Maes, M. (2013), 'So depression is an inflammatory disease, but where does the inflammation come from?'. *BMC Medicine,* 11:200.

Blondell, S.J. Hammersley-Mather, R. Veerman, J.L. (2014), 'Does physical activity prevent cognitive decline and dementia?: A systematic review and meta-analysis of longitudinal studies'. *BMC Public Health,* 14:510.

Cooney, G.M. Dwan, K. Greig, C.A. Lawlor, D.A. Rimer, J. Waugh, F.R. McMurdo, M. (2013), 'Exercise for depression'. *Cochrane Database of Systemic Reviews,* (9):CD004366. https://doi.org/10.1002/14651858.CD004366.pub6.

Curlik, D.M. Shors, T.J. (2013), 'Training your brain: Do mental and physical (MAP) training enhance cognition through the process of neurogenesis in the hippocampus?'. *Neuropharmacology,* 64(1):506–514.

Dietrich, A. McDaniel, W.F. (2004), 'Endocannabinoids and exercise'. *British Journal of Sports Medicine,* 38:536–541.

Dobson, J. Harris, C. Eadson, W. Gore, T. (2019), 'Space to thrive – A rapid evidence review of the benefits of parks and green spaces for people and communities'. https://www.greenspacescotland.org.uk/Handlers/Download. ashx?IDMF=f93b0397-3a68-486d-ac33-cf46f06e20fa [Accessed 2020].

Hamer, M. Chida, Y. (2009), 'Physical activity and risk of neurodegenerative disease: A systematic review of prospective studies'. *Psychological Medicine,* 39(1):3–11.

Klaperski, S. Koch, E. Hewel, D. Schempp, A. Müller, J. (2019), 'The influence of the exercise environment on acute stress levels and wellbeing'. *Mental Health and Prevention,* 15:200173.

Knudtson, M.D. Klein, R. Klein, B.E.K. (2006), 'Physical activity and the 15-year cumulative incidence of age-related macular degeneration: The Beaver Dam Eye Study'. *British Journal of Ophthalmology,* 90:1461–1463.

Kvam, S. Kleppe, C.L. Nordhus, I.H. Hovland, A. (2016), 'Exercise as a treatment for depression: A meta-analysis'. *Journal of Affective Disorders,* 202:67–86.

Moon, H.Y. Becke, A. Berron, D. Becker, B. Sah, N. Benoni, G. Janke, E. Lubejko, S. Greig, N. Mattison, J. Duzel, E. van Praag, H. (2016), 'Running-induced systemic Cathepsin B secretion is associated with memory function'. *Cell Metabolism,* 24(2):332–340.

Nokia, M.S. Lensu, S. Ahtiainen, J.P. Johansson, P.P. Koch, L.G. Britton, S.L. Kainulainen, H. (2016), 'Physical exercise increases adult hippocampal neurogenesis in male rats provided it is aerobic and sustained'. *Journal of Physiology,* 594(7):1855–1873.

Oppezzo, M. Schwartz, D.L. (2014), 'Give your ideas some legs: The positive effect of walking on creative thinking'. *Journal of Experimental Psychology: Learning, Memory and Cognition,* 40(4):1142–1152.

Sofi, F. Valecchi, D. Bacci, D. Abbate, R. Gensini, G.F. Casini, A. Macchi, C. (2011), 'Physical activity and risk of cognitive decline: A meta-analysis of prospective studies'. *Journal of Internal Medicine,* 269:107–117.

Tseng, V., F. Yu, and A.L. Coleman (2017), Exercise Intensity and Risk of Glaucoma in the National Health and Nutrition Examination Survey. American Academy of Ophthalmology, New Orleans, USA. https://doi.org/10.1016/j.ogla.2020.06.001.

Williams, T. (2009), 'Prospective study of incident age-related macular degeneration in relation to vigorous physical activity during a 7-year follow-up'. *Investigative Ophthalmology and Visual Science,* 50(1):101–106.

Chapter 2: The Cardiovascular System

Dayer, M.J. Green, I. (2019), 'Mortality during marathons: A narrative review of the literature'. *BMJ Open Sport and Exercise Medicine,* 5(1):e000555.

Kim, J.H. Malhotra, R. Chiampas, G. d'Hemecourt, P. Troyanos, C. Cianca, J. Smith, R.N. Wang, T.J. Roberts, W.O. Thompson, P.D. Baggish, A.L. Race Associated Cardiac Arrest Event Registry (RACER) Study Group (2012), 'Cardiac arrest during long-distance running races'. *New England Journal of Medicine,* 366(2):130–40.

La Gerche, A. Burns, A.A.T. Mooney, D.J. Inder, W.J. Taylor, A.J. Bogaert, J. MacIsaac, A.I. Heidbüchel, H. Prior, D.L. (2012), 'Exercise-induced right ventricular dysfunction and structural remodelling in endurance athletes'. *European Heart Journal,* 33(8):998–1006.

Lippi, G. Schena, F. Salvagno, G.L. Aloe, R. Banfi, G. Guidi, G.C (2012), 'Foot-strike haemolysis after a 60-km ultramarathon'. *Blood Transfusion,* 10(3):377–383.

NICE. Clinical Knowledge Summaries, 'Palpitations'. https://cks.nice.org.uk/palpitations [Accessed 2019].

NICE guidelines [NG136] (2019), 'Hypertension in adults: Diagnosis and management'. http://www.nice.org.uk/ guidance/ng136 [Accessed 2019].

Resuscitation Council (UK), 'Prehospital Resuscitation Guidelines 2015'. https://www.resus.org.uk/resuscitation-guidelines/prehospital-resuscitation/ [Accessed 2019].

Telford, R.D. Sly, G.J. Hahn, A.G. Cunningham, R.B. Bryant, C. Smith, J.A. (2003), 'Footstrike is the major cause of hemolysis during running'. *Journal of Applied Physiology,* 94(1):38–42.

Wilson, M. O'Hanlon, R. Prasad, S. Deighan, A. Macmillan, P. Oxborough, D. Godfrey, R. Smith, G. Maceira, A. Sharma, S. George, K. Whyte, G. (2011), 'Diverse patterns of myocardial fibrosis in lifelong, veteran endurance athletes'. *Journal of Applied Physiology,* 110:1622–1626.

Chapter 3: The Respiratory System

Avallone, K.M. McLeish, A.C. (2013), 'Asthma and aerobic exercise: A review of the empirical literature'. *Journal of Asthma* 50(2):109–16.

Carson, K.V. Chandratilleke, M.G. Picot, J. Brinn, M.P. Esterman, A.J. Smith, B.J. (2013), 'Physical training for asthma'. *Cochrane Database of Systematic Reviews,* (9):CD001116. https://doi.org/10.1002/14651858.CD001116.pub4.

Dallam, G.M. McClaren, S.R. Cox, D.G. Foust, C.P. (2018), 'Effect of nasal versus oral breathing on VO2 max and physiological economy in recreational runners following an extended period spent using nasally restricted breathing'. *Journal of Kinesiology and Sports Science,* 6(2):22.

Hall, A. Thomas, T. Sandhu, G. Hull, J.H. (2016), 'Exercise-induced laryngeal obstruction: A common and overlooked cause of exertional breathlessness'. *British Journal of General Practice,* 66(650): e683–e685.

Hull, J.H. (2015), 'Not all wheeze is asthma: Time for patients to exercise their rights'. *Thorax,* 70(1):7–8.

Keles, N. (2002), 'Treating allergic rhinitis in the athlete'. *Rhinology,* 40:211–214.

Molis, M.A. Molis, W.A. (2010), 'Exercise-induced Bronchospasm'. *Sports Health,* 2(4):311–317.

Parsons, J.P. Hallstrand, T.S. Mastronarde, J.G. et al. (2013), 'An official American Thoracic Society Clinical Practice Guideline: Exercise-induced Bronchoconstriction'. *American Journal of Respiratory and Critical Care Medicine,* 187:1016–27.

Recinto, R. Efthemeou, T. Boffelli, P.T. Navalta, J.W. (2017), 'Effects of nasal or oral breathing on anaerobic power output and metabolic responses'. *International Journal of Exercise Science,* 10(4):506–514.

Chapter 4: The Gastrointestinal System

Aragon, A.A. Schoenfeld, B.J. (2013), 'Nutrient timing revisited: Is there a post-exercise anabolic window?' *Journal of the International Society of Sports Nutrition,* 10:5.

British National Formulary. 'Loperamide Hydrochloride'. https://bnf.nice.org.uk/drug/loperamide-hydrochloride.html [Accessed 2019].

Ligtenberg, A.J.M. Liem, H.S. Brand, H.S. Veerman, E.C.I. (2016), 'The effect of exercise on salivary viscosity'. *Diagnostics,* 6(4):40.

Ligtenberg, A.J. Brand, H.S. van den Keijbus, P.A. Veerman, E.C. (2015), 'The effect of physical exercise on salivary secretion of MUC5B, amylase and lysozyme'. *Archives of Oral Biology,* 60(11):1639–1644.

Morton, D. Callister, R. (2015), 'Exercise-Related Transient Abdominal Pain (ETAP)'. *Sports Medicine,* 45:22–35. https://doi.org/10.1007/s40279-014-0245-z.

NICE guidelines [CG184] (2014 – updated 2019), 'Gastro-oesophageal reflux disease and dyspepsia in adults: Investigation and management'. https://www.nice.org.uk/guidance/cg184 [Accessed 2019].

NICE guidelines [NG20] (2015), 'Coeliac disease: Recognition, assessment and management'. https://www.nice.org.uk/guidance/ng20 [Accessed 2019].

Pietilä, J. Helander, E. Korhonen, I. Myllymäki, T. Kujala, UM. Lindholm, H. (2018), 'Acute effect of alcohol intake on cardiovascular autonomic regulation during the first hours of sleep in a large real-world sample of Finnish employees: Observational study'. *JMIR Mental Health,* 5(1):e23.

UK Chief Medical Officers' Low Risk Drinking Guidelines (2016), https://assets.publishing.service.gov.uk/government/uploads/system/uploads/attachment_data/file/545937/UK_CMOs__report.pdf [Accessed 2019].

Wolin, K.Y. Yan, Y. Colditz, G.A. Lee, I.M. (2009), 'Physical activity and colon cancer prevention: A meta-analysis'. *British Journal of Cancer,* 100, 611–616.

Chapter 5: The Urinary System

Alhazmi, H.H. (2015), 'Microscopic haematuria in athletes: A review of the literature'. *Saudi Journal of Sports Medicine,* 15(2):131–136.

Almond, C.S.D. et al. (2005), 'Hyponatremia among runners in the Boston Marathon'. *New England Journal of Medicine,* 352:1550–1556.

Bally, M. Dendukiuri, N. Rich, B. Nadeau, L. Helin-Salmivaara, A. Garbe, E. Brophy, J.M. (2017), 'Risk of acute myocardial infarction with NSAIDs in real world use: Bayesian meta-analysis of individual patient data'. *British Medical Journal,* 357:j1909.

Benke, I.L. Leitzmann, M.F. Behrens, G. Schmid, D. (2018), 'Physical activity in relation to risk of prostate cancer: A systematic review and meta-analysis'. *Annals of Oncology,* 29(5):1154–1179.

Clarkson, P.M. (2007), 'Exertional rhabdomyolysis and acute renal failure in marathon runners'. *Sports Medicine,* 37(4–5):361–363.

Hewing, B. Schattke, S. Spethmann, S. Sanad, W. Schroeckh, S. Schimke, I. Halleck, F. Peters, H. Brechtel, L. Lock, J. Baumann, G. Dreger, H. Borges, A.C. Knebel, F. (2015), 'Cardiac and renal function in a large cohort of amateur marathon runners'. *Cardiovascular Ultrasound,* Mar 21;13:13.

Jones, G.R. Newhouse, I. (1997), 'Sport related haematuria: A review'. *Clinical Journal of Sport Medicine,* 7(2):119–125.

Kao, W.F. Hou, S.K. Chiu, Y.H. Chou, S.L. Kuo, F.C. Wang, S.H. Chen, J.J (2015), 'Effects of 100-km ultramarathon on acute kidney injury'. *Clinical Journal of Sport Medicine,* 25(1): 49–54.

Kipps, C. Sharma, S. Pedoe, D.T. (2011), 'The incidence of exercise-associated hyponatraemia in the London marathon'. *British Journal of Sports Medicine,* 45:14–19.

Lipman, G.S. Krabak, B.J. Rundell, S.D Shea, K.M. Badowski, N. Little, C. (2016), 'Incidence and prevalence of acute kidney injury during multistage ultramarathons'. *Clinical Journal of Sport Medicine* 26(4):314–319.

Lipman, G.S. Shea, K. Christensen, M. et al. (2017), 'Ibuprofen versus placebo effect on acute kidney injury in ultramarathons: A randomised controlled trial'. *Emergency Medicine Journal,* 34:637–642.

Luthje, P. Nurmi, I. (2004), 'Recurrent macroscopic haematuria due to bladder blood vessels after exercise induced haematuria'. *British Journal of Sports Medicine,* 38:e4.

Mansour, S.G. Verma, G. Pata, R.W. Martin, T.G Perazella, M.A. Parikh, C.R. (2017), 'Kidney injury and repair biomarkers in marathon runners'. *American Journal of Kidney Diseases,* 70(2):252–261.

Millman, A.L. Cheung, C.D. Hackett, C. Elterman, D. (2018), 'Overactive bladder in men: A practical approach'. *British Journal of General Practice,* 68(671):298–299.

Siegel, A.J. Hennekens, M.D. Solomon, H.S (1979), 'Exercise-related haematuria. Findings in a group of marathon runners'. *Journal of the American Medical Association,* 241(4):391–392.

Silva, V. Grande, A.J. Peccin, M.S (2019), 'Physical activity for lower urinary tract symptoms secondary to benign prostatic obstruction'. *Cochrane Database of Systematic Reviews,* (4):CD012044. https://doi.org/10.1002/14651858.CD012044. pub2.

Varma, P.P. Sengupta, P. Nair, R.K (2014), 'Post exertional hematuria'. *Renal Failure,* 36(5):701–703.

Williams, P.T. (2008), 'Effects of running distance and performance on incident benign prostatic hyperplasia'. *Medicine and Science in Sports and Exercise,* 40(10):1733–1739.

Chapter 6: The Reproductive System

Arce, J.M. De Souza, M.J. (1993), 'Exercise and male factor infertility'. *Sports Medicine,* 15(3):146–169.

Asikainen, T.M. Kukkonen-Harjula, K. Miilunpalo, S. (2004), 'Exercise for health for early postmenopausal women: A systematic review of randomised controlled trials'. *Sports Medicine,* 34(11):753–778.

Bailey T.G., Cable N.T., Aziz N., Atkinson G., Cuthbertson D.J., Low D.A., Jones H. (2016), 'Exercise training reduces the acute physiological severity of post-menopausal hot flushes'. *Journal of Physiology – London,* 594:657–667.

Boone, T. Gilmore, S. (1995), 'Effects of sexual intercourse on maximal aerobic power, oxygen pulse and double product in male sedentary subjects'. *Journal of Sports Medicine and Physical Fitness,* 35(3):214–217.

Bruinvels, G. Burden, R. Brown, N. Richards, T. Pedlar, C (2016), 'The prevalence and impact of heavy menstrual bleeding (menorrhagia) in elite and non-elite athletes'. *PLoS ONE,* 11(2):e0149881.

Bruinvels, G. Burden, R.J. McGregor, A.J. Ackerman, K. E. Dooley, M. Richards, T. Pedlar, C. (2017), 'Sport, exercise and the menstrual cycle: Where is the research?' *British Journal of Sports Medicine,* 51(6):487–488.

Carey, G.B. Quinn, T.J. (2001), 'Exercise and lactation: Are they compatible?' *Canadian Journal of Applied Physiology,* 26(1):55–75.

Daley, A. Stokes-Lampard, H. Thomas, A. MacArthur, C. (2014), 'Exercise for vasomotor menopausal symptoms'. *Cochrane Database of Systematic Reviews,* Nov28;(11):CD006108. https://doi.org/10.1002/14651858.CD006108.pub4

Daley, A. Thomas, A. Cooper, H. Fitzpatrick, H. McDonald, C. Moore, H. Rooney, R. Deeks, J.J. (2012, 'Maternal exercise and growth in breastfed infants: A meta-analysis of randomized controlled trials'. *Pediatrics,* 130(1):108–114.

Dunson, D. Colombo, B. Baird, D.D. (2002), 'Changes with age in the level and duration of fertility in the menstrual cycle'. *Human Reproduction,* 17(5):1399–1403.

Fergus, K.B. Gaither, T.W. Baradaran, N. Glidden, D.V. Cohen, A.J. Breyer, B.N. (2019), 'Exercise improves self-reported sexual function among physically active adults'. *Journal of Sexual Medicine,* 16(8):1236–1245.

Goom, T. Donnelly, G. Brockwell, E. (2019) 'Ready, steady...GO! Ensuring postnatal women are run-ready!' https://blogs.bmj.com/bjsm/2019/05/20/ready-steadygo-ensuring-postnatal-women-are-run-ready/ [Accessed 2019].

Hajizadeh Maleki, B. Tartibian, B. (2015), 'Long-term low-to-intensive cycling training: Impact on semen parameters and seminal cytokines'. *Clinical Journal of Sports Medicine,* 25(6):535–540.

Hajizadeh Maleki, B. Tartibian, B. Chehrazi, M. (2017), 'The effects of three different exercise modalities on markers of male reproduction in healthy subjects: A randomized controlled trial'. *Reproduction,* 153(2):157–174.

Janse de Jonge, X.A. (2003), 'Effects of the menstrual cycle on exercise performance'. *Sports Medicine,* 33(11):833–851.

Jóźków, P. Rossato, M. (2017), 'The impact of intense exercise on semen quality'. *American Journal of Men's Health,* 11(3):654–662.

Lumsden, M.A. Gebbie, A. Holland, C. (2013), 'Managing unscheduled bleeding in non-pregnant premenopausal women'. *British Medical Journal,* 346:f3251.

Masour, D. (2017), 'Postponing menstruation: Choices and concerns'. *Journal of Family Planning and Reproductive Health Care,* 43:160–161.

McGlone, S. Shrier, I. (2000), 'Does sex the night before competition decrease performance?' *Clinical Journal of Sport Medicine,* 10(4):233–234.

NICE. Clinical Knowledge Summaries (2019), 'Amenorrhoea'. https://cks.nice.org.uk/amenorrhoea [Accessed 2020].

Oosthuyuse, T. Bosch, A.N. (2010), 'The effect of the menstrual cycle on exercise metabolism: Implications for exercise performance in eumenorrhoeic women'. *Sports Medicine,* 40(3):207–227.

Quinn, T.J. Carey, G.B. (1999) 'Does exercise intensity or diet influence lactic acid accumulation in breast milk?' *Medicine and Science in Sports and Exercise,* 31(1):105–110.

Stefani, L. Galanti, G. Padulo, J. Bragazzi, N.L. Maffulli, N. (2016), 'Sexual activity before sports competition: A systematic review'. *Frontiers in Physiology* 7:246.

Su, D. Zhao, Z. Binns, C. Scott, J. Oddy, W. (2007), 'Breast-feeding mothers can exercise: Results of a cohort study'. *Public Health Nutrition,* 10(10):1089–1093.

The American College of Obstetrics and Gynecologists Committee Opinion (2020), 'Physical activity and exercise during pregnancy and the postpartum period'. https://www.acog.org/clinical/clinical-guidance/committee-opinion/articles/2020/04/physical-activity-and-exercise-during-pregnancy-and-the-postpartum-period [Accessed 2020]

Wallace, J.P. Rabin, J. (1991) 'The concentration of lactic acid in breast milk following maximal exercise'. *International Journal of Sports Medicine* 12(3):328–331.

Whincup, P.H. Gilg, J.A. Odoki, K. Taylir, S.J.C. Cook, D.G (2001), 'Age of menarche in contemporary British teenagers: Survey of girls born between 1982 and 1986'. *British Medical Journal,* 322:1095.

Wright, K.S. Quinn, T.J. Carey, G.B. (2002) 'Infant acceptance of breast milk after maternal exercise'. *Pediatrics,* 109(4):585–589.

Zavorsky, G.S. Vouyoukas, E. Pfaus, J.G. (2019), 'Sexual activity the night before exercise does not affect various measures of physical exercise performance'. *Sexual Medicine,* 7(2):235–240.

Chapter 7: The Musculoskeletal System

Alexander, J.L.N. Barton, C.J. Willy, R.W. (2019), 'Infographic. Running myth: Static stretching reduces injury risk in runners'. *British Journal of Sports Medicine Online First.* https://doi.org/10.1136/bjsports-2019-101169.

Alexander, J.L.N. Barton, C.J. Willy, R.W. (2019), 'Infographic. Running myth: Strength training should be high repetition low load to improve running performance'. *British Journal of Sports Medicine Online First.* https://doi.org/10.1136/bjsports-2019-101168.

American College of Sports Medicine (2011), 'Delayed onset muscle soreness'. http://www.acsm.org/docs/default-source/files-for-resource-library/delayed-onset-muscle-soreness-(doms).pdf [Accessed 2019]

Babtunde, O.O. Jordan, J.L. van der Windt, D.A. Hill, J.C. Foster, N.E. Protheroe, J. (2017), 'Effective treatment options for musculoskeletal pain in primary care: A systematic overview of current evidence'. *PloS One,* 12(6):e0178621.

Barton, C.J. Lack, S. Malliaras, P. Morrissey, D. (2013), 'Gluteal muscle activity and patellofemoral pain syndrome: A systematic review'. *British Journal of Sports Medicine,* 47(4):207–214.

Bates, P. (1985). 'Shin splints: A literature review'. *British Journal of Sports Medicine,* 19:132–137.

Chakravarty, E.F. Hubert, H.B. Lingala, V.B. Zatarain, E. Fries, J.F. (2008), 'Long distance running and knee osteoarthritis. A prospective study'. *American Journal of Preventative Medicine,* 35(2):133–138.

Cheng, Y. Macera, C.A. Davis, D.R. Ainsworth, B.E. Troped, P.J. Blair, S.N. (2000), 'Physical activity and self-reported, physician-diagnosed osteoarthritis: Is physical activity a risk factor?' *Journal of Clinical Epidemiology,* 53(3):315–322.

Coggon, D. Reading, I. Croft, P. Barrett, D. Cooper, C. (2001), 'Knee osteoarthritis and obesity'. *International Journal of Obesity and Related Metabolic Disorders,* 25(5):622–627.

Cymet, T.C. Sinkov, V. (2006), 'Does long-distance running cause osteoarthritis?' *Journal of the American Osteopathic Association,* 106(6):342–345.

Dupuy, O. Douzi, W. Theurot, D. Bosquet, L. Dugué, B. (2018), 'An evidence-based approach for choosing post-exercise recovery techniques to reduce markers of muscle damage, soreness, fatigue and inflammation: A systematic review with meta-analysis'. *Frontiers in Physiology,* 9:403.

Earl, J.E. Hoch, A.Z. (2011), 'A proximal strengthening program improves pain, function and biomechanics in women with patellofemoral pain syndrome'. *American Journal of Sports Medicine,* 39(1):154–163.

Ernst, E. (1998), 'Does post-exercise massage treatment reduce delayed onset muscle soreness? A systematic review'. *British Journal of Sports Medicine,* 32:212–214.

Fransen, M. McConnell, S. (2008), 'Exercise for osteoarthritis of the knee'. *Cochrane Database of Systematic Reviews* (4):CD004376. https://doi.org/10.1002/14651858.CD004376.pub2.

Hill, J. Howatson, G. van Someron, K. Leeder, J. Pedlar, C. (2013), 'Compression garments and recovery from exercise-induced muscle damage: A meta-analysis'. *British Journal of Sports Medicine Online First.* https://doi.org/10.1136/bjsports-2013-092456.

Horga, L.M. Henckel, J. Fotiadou et al. (2019), 'Can marathon running improve knee damage of middle-aged adults? A prospective cohort study'. *BMJ Open Sport and Exercise Medicine,* 5:e000586.

Kerhoffs, G.M. van den Bekerom, M. Elders, L.A.M. et al. (2012), 'Diagnosis, treatment and prevention of ankle sprains: An evidence-based clinical guideline'. *British Journal of Sports Medicine,* 46:859–865.

Khaled, A.A. (2017), 'Gender disparities in osteoporosis'. *Journal of Clinical Medicine Research,* 9(5):382–387.

Kujala, U.M. Sarna, S. Kaprio, J. Tikkanen, H.O. Koskenvuo, M. (2000), 'Natural selection to sports, later physical activity habits, and coronary heart disease'. *British Journal of Sports Medicine,* 34:445–449.

Larson, P. Higgins, E. Kaminski, J. Decker, T. Preble, J. Lyons, D. McIntyre, K. Normile, A. (2011), 'Foot strike patterns of recreational and sub-elite runners in a long-distance road race'. *Journal of Sports Sciences,* 28(15):1665–1673.

Li, Y. Su, Y. Chen, S. Zhang, S. Liu, C Lu, M. Liu, F. Li, S. He, Z. Wang, Y. Sheng, L. Wang, W. Zhan, Z. Wang, X. Zheng, N. (2016), 'The effects of resistance exercise in patients with knee osteoarthritis: A systematic review and meta-analysis'. *Clinical Rehabilitation,* 30(10):947–959.

Luedke, L.E. Heiderscheit, B.C. Williams, D.S. Rauh, M.J. (2016), 'Influence of step rate on shin injury and anterior knee pain in high school runners'. *Medicine and Science in Sport and Exercise,* 48(7):1244–1250.

Ly, M. Fitzpatrick, J. Ellis, B. Loftis, T. (2019), 'Why are musculoskeletal conditions the biggest contributor to morbidity'. *Health Profile for England,* https://publichealthmatters.blog.gov.uk/2019/03/11/why-are-musculoskeletal-conditions-the-biggest-contributor-to-morbidity/ [Accessed 2020].

Mattacola, C.G. Dwyer, M.K. (2002), 'Rehabilitation of the ankle after acute sprain or chronic instability'. *Journal of Athletic Training,* 37(4):413–429.

NICE. Clinical Knowledge Summaries. 'Morton's neuroma'. https://cks.nice.org.uk/mortons-neuroma [Accessed 2019].

Nilwik, R. Snijders, T. Leenders, M. Groen, B.B. van Kranenburg, J. Verdijk, L.B. van Loon, L.J. (2013), 'The decline in skeletal muscle mass with aging is mainly attributed to a reduction in type II muscle fibre size'. *Experimental Gerontology,* 48(5):492–498.

Noehren, B. Scholz, J. Davis, I. (2011), 'The effect of real-time gait retraining on hip kinematics, pain and function in subjects with patellofemoral pain syndrome'. *British Journal of Sports Medicine,* 45:691–696.

Pearcey, G.E. Bradbury-Squires, D.J. Kawamoto, J.E. Drinkwater, E.J. Behm, D.G. Button, D.C. (2015), 'Foam rolling for delayed-onset muscle soreness and recovery of dynamic performance measures'. *Journal of Athletic Training,* 50(1):5–13.

Pegrum, J. Self, A. Hall, N. (2019), 'Iliotibial band syndrome'. *British Medical Journal,* 364:1980.

Quicke, J.G. Foster, N.E. Thomas, M.J. Holden, M.A. (2015), 'Is long-term physical activity safe for older adults with knee pain?: A systematic review'. *Osteoarthritis Cartilage,* 23(9):1445–1456.

Romani, W.A. Gieck, J.H. Perrin, D.H. Saliba, E.N. Kahler, D.M. (2002), 'Mechanisms and management of stress fractures in physically active persons'. *Journal of Athletic Training,* 37(3):306–314.

Rønnestad, B.R. Mujika, I. (2013), 'Optimizing strength training for running and cycling endurance performance: A review'. *Scandinavian Journal of Medicine and Science in Sport,* 24(4):603–612.

Schroeder, A.N. Best, T.M. (2015), 'Is self myofascial release an effective preexercise and recovery strategy? A literature review'. *Current Sports Medicine Reports,* 14(3):200–208.

Schwellnus, M.P. (2009), 'Cause of Exercise Associated Muscle Cramps (EAMC) – altered neuromuscular control, dehydration or electrolyte depletion?' *British Journal of Sports Medicine,* 43:401–408.

Stecco, C. Corradin, M. Macchi, V. Morra, A. Porzionato, A. Biz, C. De Caro, R. (2013), 'Plantar fascia anatomy and its relationship with Achilles tendon and paratenon'. *Journal of Anatomy,* 223(6):665–676.

Wilson, J.M. Loenneke, J.P. Jo, E. Wilso, G.J. Zourdos, M.C. Kim, J.S. (2012), 'The effects of endurance, strength and power training on muscle fibre type shifting'. *Journal of Strength and Conditioning Research,* 26(6):1724–1729.

Timmins, K.A. Leech, R.D. Batt, M.E. Edwards, K.L. (2017), 'Running and knee osteoarthritis: A systematic review and meta-analysis'. *The American Journal of Sports Medicine,* 45(6):1447–1457.

Uthman, O.A. Jordan, J.L. van der Windt, D.A. Dziedzic, K.S. Healey, E.L. Peat, G.M. Foster, N.E. (2013), 'Exercise for lower limb osteoarthritis: Systematic review incorporating trial sequential analysis and network meta-analysis'. *British Medical Journal,* 346:f5555. https://doi.org/10.1136/bmj.f5555.

Winters, M. Bon, P. Bijvoet, E.W.P. Moen, M.H. (2017), 'Are ultrasonographic findings like periosteal and tendinous edema associated with medial tibial stress syndrome? A case-control study'. *Journal of Science and Medicine in Sport,* 20(2):128–133.

Wright, A.A. Taylor, J.B. Ford, K.R. Siska, L. Smoliga, J.M. (2015), 'Risk factors associated with lower extremity stress fractures in runners: A systematic review with meta-analysis'. *British Journal of Sports Medicine,* 49:1517–1523.

Vasiliadis, A. (2017), 'Common stress fractures in runners: An analysis'. *Saudi Journal of Sports Medicine,* 17(1):1–6.

Zügel, M. Maganaris, C.N. Wilke et al. (2018), 'Fascial tissue research in sports medicine: From molecules to tissue adaptation, injury and diagnostics: Consensus statement'. *British Journal of Sports Medicine*, 52:1497.

Chapter 8: The Skin

Crawford, F. Hollis, S. (2007), 'Topical treatments for fungal infections of the skin and nails of the foot'. *Cochrane Database of Systematic Reviews*, (3):CD001434. https://doi.org/10.1002/14651858.CD001434.pub2.

NICE. Clinical Knowledge Summaries, 'Paronychia – acute'. https://cks.nice.org.uk/paronychia-acute [Accessed 2020].

NICE. Clinical Knowledge Summaries, 'Urticaria'. https://cks.nice.org.uk/urticaria [Accessed 2020].

NICE. Clinical Knowledge Summaries, 'Warts and Verrucae'. https://cks.nice.org.uk/warts-and-verrucae [Accessed 2020].

Chapter 9: Self-Care

Budgett, R. (1998), 'Fatigue and underperformance in athletes: The overtraining syndrome'. *British Journal of Sports Medicine*, 32:107–110.

Carter, D. Amblum-Almer, J. (2015), 'Analgesia for people with acute ankle sprain'. *Emergency Nurse*, 23(1):24–31.

Fradkin, A.J. Gabbe, B.J. Cameron, P.A. (2006), 'Does warming up prevent injury in sport? The evidence from randomised controlled trials'. *Journal of Science and Medicine in Sport*, 9(3):214–220.

Keimling, M. Behrens, G. Schmid, D. Jochem, C. Leitzmann, M.F. (2014), 'The association between physical activity and bladder cancer: Systematic review and meta-analysis'. *British Journal of Cancer*, 110(7):1862–70.

Lipman, G.S. Gaudio, F.G. Eifling, K.P. Ellis, M.A. Otten, E.M. Grissom, C.K. (2019), 'Wilderness Medical Society Clinical Practice Guidelines for the Prevention and Treatment of Heat Illness: 2019 Update'. *Wilderness and Environmental Medicine*, 30(4):S22–46.

Meeusen, R. Duclos, M. Foster, C. Fry, A. Gleeson, M. Nieman, D. Raglin, J. Rietjens, G. Steinacker, J. Urhausen, A. (2013), 'Prevention, diagnosis, and treatment of the overtraining syndrome: Joint consensus statement of the European College of Sport Science and the American College of Sports Medicine'. *Medicine and Science in Sports and Exercise*, 45(1):186–205.

Montgomery, P. Dennis, J.A. (2002), 'Physical exercise for sleep problems in adults aged 60+'. *Cochrane Database of Systemic Reviews*, (4):CD003404. https://doi.org/10.1002/14651858.CD003404.

Neilson, H.K. Farris, M.S. Stone, C.R. Vaska, M.M. Friedenreich, C.M. (2017), 'Moderate-vigorous recreational physical activity and breast cancer risk, stratified by menopause status: A systematic review and meta-analysis'. *Menopause*, 24(3):322–344.

NHS 'Heat exhaustion and heatstroke'. https://www.nhs.uk/conditions/heat-exhaustion-heatstroke/ [Accessed 2020].

NICE. Clinical Knowledge Summaries (2015), 'Insomnia'. https://cks.nice.org.uk/insomnia [Accessed 2020].

NICE. Clinical Knowledge Summaries (2015), 'Sprains and strains'. http://cks.nice.org.uk/sprains-and-strains [Accessed 2020].

Orchard, J. Best, T.M. (2002), 'The management of muscle strain injuries: An early return versus the risk of recurrence'. *Clinical Journal of Sport Medicine,* 13:3–5.

Pedersen, B.K. Toft, A.D. (2000), 'Effects of exercise on lymphocytes and cytokines'. *British Journal of Sports Medicine,* 34:246–251.

Pijpe, A. Manders, P. Brohet, R.M. Colleé, J.M. Verhoef, S. Vasen, H.F. Hoogerbrugge, N. van Asperen, C.J. Dommering, C. Ausems, M.G. Aalfs, C.M. Gomez-Garcia, E.B. Hebon, Van't Leer, L.J. van Leeuwen, F.E. Rookus, M.A. (2010), 'Physical activity and the risk of breast cancer in BRCA ½ mutation carriers'. *Breast Cancer Research and Treatment,* 120(1):235–244.

Siegel, R. Laursen, P.B. (2012), 'Keeping your cool: Possible mechanisms for enhanced exercise performance in the heat with internal cooling methods'. *Sports Medicine,* 42(2):89–98.

UK Chief Medical Officers' Physical Activity Guidelines (2019), https://assets.publishing.service.gov.uk/government/uploads/system/uploads/attachment_data/file/832868/uk-chief-medical-officers-physical-activity-guidelines.pdf [Accessed 2020].

van Mechelen, W. (1992), 'Running injuries. A review of the epidemiological literature'. *Sports Medicine,* 14(5):320–335.

van Poppel, D. de Koning, J. Verhagen, A.P. Scholten-Peeters, G.G. (2016), 'Risk factors for lower extremity injuries among half marathon and marathon runners of the Lage Landen Marathon Eindhoven 2012: A prospective cohort study in the Netherlands'. *Scandinavian Journal of Medicine and Science in Sports,* 26(2):226–234.

Whiteman, D.C. Wilson, L.F. (2016), 'The fractions of cancer attributable to modifiable factors: A global review'. *Cancer Epidemiology,* 44:203–221.

Wilber, R.L. Moffatt, R.J. (1994), 'Physiological and biochemical consequences of detraining in aerobically trained individuals'. *The Journal of Strength and Conditioning Research,* 8(2):110–124.

INDEX

abscesses 187
Achilles tendon 156–7, 160, 161–2
acid reflux 69, 70, 85
acne 195
actinic keratoses 182
addiction, running 7–8
adrenal glands 89
adrenalin 63, 74, 76, 220
age-related macular degeneration (AMD) 25
airways 51, 59
alcohol 34, 69, 75, 79–82, 85, 104, 115, 149, 153, 220
aldosterone 89
allergies 22, 54–5, 63, 77, 190
alveoli 49–50, 51
Alzheimer's disease 10, 11
ambulatory blood pressure monitoring (ABPM) 32
amenorrhoea 121–2, 124, 218
anaemia 20, 34, 39–41, 120, 121, 125, 219
anal sphincter 76
anaphylaxis 190
aneurysms 25
ankles, sprained 162–3
antacid medications 69
anti-bacterial wash 195
anti-diarrhoea tablets 76–7
anti-fungal tablets 192
anti-inflammatory effect, exercise 5, 216
anti-inflammatory medication 69, 94–5, 97, 107, 121, 157, 162
antibiotics 106, 187, 192, 197
antidepressants 16–18, 77
antihistamines 22, 53, 54, 190
antiperspirants 198
anxiety 18–19, 20, 30, 35, 112, 113
aorta 29, 64
apocrine glands 198
apps 30, 220
arm muscles 139
arthritis 142, 143, 144–6, 154, 155
asthma 55–8
athlete's foot/tinea pedis 184, 192, 193
atria 29, 47
atrial fibrillation (AF) 34, 47, 81
automated external defibrillators (AED) 45–6

balance 4, 20, 81, 127, 228–9
barrier creams 185, 199
basal cell carcinoma (BCC) 182–3
belonging, sense of 5–6
benign prostatic hypertrophy (BPH) 102–3
biomechanics 142, 151, 157, 158, 162, 168
bladder, the 89, 95, 101–2, 103–4, 105–6, 107
blisters 178–80
blood 29–30
    donation 37–8
    loss 39

peeing 95–7, 106
in poo/from back passage 77, 85
blood pressure 4, 11, 20, 23, 24, 28, 32–3, 37, 42, 47, 89, 91, 93, 94, 107, 113, 124
blood sugar levels 23, 33, 42, 80, 81
blurred vision 21–3
body awareness 41, 47, 126, 127
body fat 5, 71, 194, 216–17
bone anatomy 134
bone health 131, 140, 146–51
bone marrow 39, 134
bowels 74, 75, 76, 77, 84, 85, 101, 102
brain anatomy 3–4
brain-derived neurotrophic factor (BDNF) 9
brain training 9
bras, sports 174–5, 177
breastfeeding 129–30
breasts 126, 132, 176–7
breathing techniques 4, 12, 52, 59, 72, 73, 75
breathlessness 43, 202
bronchi 49, 57
buttock pain 164–5, 166

cadence, running 148, 161
caffeine 34, 104, 130, 220, 221
calamine lotion 190
calf muscles 149, 157, 161, 162
cancer 39, 66, 70, 84, 85, 95, 96, 102, 103, 123, 182–3, 206–7, 216, 228
caps and visors 181, 197, 222
carbon dioxide expulsion 49, 50, 64
cardiac arrest see heart attacks
cardiac remodelling 46
cardiovascular disease 30, 43
cardiovascular system 28, 218
    see also heart
cartilage 139, 143
cathepsin B (CTSB) 9
cellulite 194
cervical ectropion 123
cervical smear tests 123–4, 132
cervical spine 166–7
chafed skin 174–6
chest compressions 45
chest muscles 51, 59
chest pains 35–6, 43, 60
chewing properly 74, 75, 85
chilblains 177–8
childbirth 97, 99, 107, 128–9, 132
chronic kidney disease (CKD) 93
circulation 28–9, 36, 114, 136, 177, 178
clothing 36, 37, 54, 55, 56, 98, 116, 136, 162, 174–7, 179, 189, 191, 193, 196, 197, 199, 222, 225, 229
    see also shoes, running
co-ordination 4, 228–9
coeliac disease 82–3
cognitive function 10

cold air/weather   26, 53, 63, 68, 225–6
cold fingers   36, 225
colds   60, 63, 201, 202–4
commensals   185
compression garments   37, 116, 136, 162
conceiving and running   124
constipation   66, 74, 76, 77, 84, 85, 98, 99, 102
cool downs/warm downs   33, 47, 56, 71
Cooper's ligaments   176
core strength   139, 151, 152, 169, 214
corneal abrasion   22–3
coronary heart disease   28, 138
coughing   57, 60, 98, 99
counselling   17
CPR (cardiopulmonary resuscitation)   45
cramps   136–7, 223
Crohn's disease   83–4
cystitis   105–6

dehydration   20, 25, 33, 57, 68, 70–1, 78, 80,
     81, 90, 93, 95, 97, 136, 137
  see also hydration
delayed onset muscle soreness (DOMS)   135–6
dementia   10–11
depression   16–18, 30, 113, 129
dermis   172, 173, 198
diabetes   23, 24, 42, 93, 94, 104, 113, 124,
     126, 136, 137, 153, 177, 189, 206
diaphragm   51, 72
diaphragmatic breathing   52, 59, 64
diarrhoea   74–7, 78, 79
diastolic blood pressure   32
diet/nutrition   37, 40, 41, 47, 64, 70, 71,
     73–4, 75, 78, 82, 84–5, 107, 124, 130, 132,
     150, 170, 194, 197, 199, 201, 203, 204, 213,
     215–16, 217–18, 229
digestion   66, 68, 70, 72, 74, 75, 218
dip stick urine tests   95, 96
dizziness   20–1, 33, 34, 63, 77, 124, 202, 223
donating blood   37–8
drinking see alcohol; dehydration; hydration
dry eyes   22
dynamic stretches   138–9, 170, 227

ears   20–1
eating disorders   218
eating on the move   73, 76
eccrine glands   198
eczema   196
ejaculation   100, 102
electrocardiogram (ECG)   34
electrolytes   91, 107, 223
elevating body parts   33, 37, 163, 209
emergencies, medical   23–4, 25, 34, 35,
     44–5, 190
emollients   196
endocannabinoids   7
endorphins   5, 6, 7
endurance athletics   7, 39–40, 46–7, 94,
     137, 138
energy levels, low   219–20
epidermis   172–3, 178
epilepsy   206
epithelial cells   173, 174
erectile dysfunction   100, 113, 114
exercise-induced asthma/bronchospasm
     (EIA/EIB)   57–8

exercise induced laryngeal obstruction
     (EILO)   58
exercise-induced orgasms   114
extracorporeal shock wave therapy   157
eyes   21–5, 54

face sag   183
faecal incontinence   99, 107, 128–9
fascia   141, 156–7
fast-twitch fibres   137, 138
feet
  athlete's foot   184, 192, 193
  causes of pain   154–5
  foot strengthening exercises   155–6, 169
  Morton's neuroma   153, 155, 158–9
  pins and needles in   152–3
  plantar fasciitis   154, 156–8
  toe nails   191–3
  verruca   188–9
fertility   114–15, 218
fibre, dietary   85
fibroids   123
fingers, white   36
first aid   44–5, 162
fitness levels, dropping   213–14
floaters   23
foam rolling   140–1, 162, 168
folic acid   124
food diaries   73–4, 75, 85
food poisoning   78–9
foot strikes
  changing   160–1
  haemolysis   39
  timing   73
  types of   159–61
fractures, stress   150–1, 155
freeze sprays   188–9
friends and support   5, 15, 19, 27, 75, 125, 206
fungal infections   184–6, 191–3

gait, running   142, 149, 152, 168, 169
gas   73–4, 83
gastro oesophageal reflux disease
     (GORD)   69–70
gastrointestinal system, anatomy of   66–8
genetics   37, 42, 43, 61, 84, 137, 142, 183,
     198, 211
gestational diabetes   124, 126
glaucoma   24
glomerulus   87, 89, 95
gloves   36, 54, 178, 226
glucose levels   80, 81
glute muscles   98, 139, 140, 151, 169, 212
gluten   82–3
glycogen stores   71, 80
goal setting   5, 113
Golgi tendon organs   136–7
greater trochanteric pain syndrome
     (GTPS)   169–70
guide runners   24
guilt, exercise   11–12
gut bacteria/microbiome   68, 85

haemoglobin   38, 39–40
haemorrhoids   84–5
hair follicles   187, 198
hangovers   81

hay fever, managing 54–5
headaches 25–6, 63, 77, 223
heart 20, 28, 30, 47
  anatomy 29–30, 35
  attacks 35, 42, 43, 44–5, 94
  beat 33
  block 34
  chest pains 35–6
  damage from running 46–7
  disease 34, 42, 138, 228
  palpitations 34–5
  rate 30, 31, 41, 51, 201, 202
heartburn 69, 70
heat cramps 223
heat rash 189–90
heat stroke/exhaustion 70, 223–5
heavy periods 120–1
heel bone/calcaneus 161
heel lock lacing 180–1
heel pads 157
heel striking 159–60, 161, 167
hernias 70, 116–17
high blood pressure 24, 32–3, 42, 91, 93–4,
  107, 113, 114, 124
hips 139, 151, 164–5, 167–8, 169–70
hives 190
homeostasis 200
hormonal contraceptives 119, 120, 123
hormones 4, 89, 97, 110, 111, 119, 130
  changes 34, 37, 107, 221
hot weather 26, 94, 97, 222–3
hydration 33, 70, 71, 72, 75, 80, 81, 83, 84,
  85, 87, 90, 91–2, 106, 107, 126, 130, 190,
  199, 203, 223
  see also dehydration
hyperhidrosis 198
hypertrophic cardiomyopathy (HOCM) 43
hypodermis 172, 173
hypoglycaemic attacks 23
hyponatraemia 70, 91–2, 222

ibuprofen 69, 94–5, 148, 157, 210–11
ice 136, 157, 162, 169, 209, 223
iliotibial band syndrome (ITBS) 167–9, 212
immune function/system 80, 182–3, 200–1,
  202, 203, 204, 218
incontinence 97–100, 102, 107, 128–9
indigestion 35, 127
inflammation 5, 57, 63, 84, 168, 169, 197,
  210, 216–17
ingrown toe nails 193
inhalers, asthma 56, 57, 58
injuries, running and 208–14, 229
insomnia 220–1
intelligence 8–9
intermenstrual bleeding 123
intestines 67, 68, 82
iron levels 37, 38–41, 96, 120, 137
irregular pulse 34
irritable bowel syndrome (IBS) 77–8

jock itch 185
joints 134, 139, 142–5, 162–3

Kegels 99
kidneys, the 87, 89, 91, 93–5, 97, 106
  damage 93–5, 107

knees
  iliotibial band 167–8
  joints 139, 142–3, 144–6, 159
  runner's knee 151–2

lacing your shoes 153, 179, 180–1
lactic acid 129, 135
leaking urine 97–8
leptin and ghrelin 71
ligaments 134, 160, 162–3, 176–7, 208
liver, the 79
loperamide 76–7
lubricants, protective 175, 176, 178, 179, 222
lungs 28, 35, 49–51, 55, 56, 60

macular degeneration 25
marathon deaths 43
marathons and kidney damage 93–4
massage 141, 168
maximum heart rate 31
medial tibial stress syndrome 147–8
melanocytes 173
melanomas 182, 183
memory function 9, 10
menisci 145
menopause 34, 37, 97, 104, 122, 130, 131,
  149, 221
menstrual cycle 118–22, 124, 132
menstruation 39, 95, 111, 119–22
mental health 5, 16–17, 55, 113, 126, 131
metatarsalgia 154–5, 158
microscopic haematuria 95–6
migraines/migraine auras 23, 26
mindful running 12
mineral levels 136
miscarriages 124, 125–6
mitochondria 134
moisturisers 183, 196
moles 182, 199
mood swings 131, 223
Morton's neuroma 153, 155, 158–9
motivation 14–15
mouth breathing 52, 68
mucous 53, 60, 63, 68
muscles 5, 9, 28, 33, 61
  abdominal 128, 129
  airways 51, 57
  anatomy of 134
  bladder/detrusor 89
  calf 149, 157, 161, 162
  chest 51, 59
  cramps 136–7
  diaphragm 59, 72
  differences in fast and slow running
    137–8
  foam rolling 140–1
  foot pain 154
  increasing mass 216–17
  injured 208
  leg and hip 37, 152, 167–8
  pain/DOMS 135–6
  perimenopause and menopause 131
  piriformis syndrome 164–5
  skeletal 28, 70, 80, 95
  sphincter 66–7, 69, 76, 89
  strength and conditioning work 139–40,
    227–8, 229

stretching 138-9
see also glutes; heart; pelvic floor
musculoskeletal system, anatomy of 133-5
see also muscles
myocardial fibrosis 46-7
myocytes 134
myoglobinuria 97
myokines 5, 9, 216

nasal breathing 52
nausea 34, 60, 71, 76-7
neck pain 166-7
nephrons 87-8, 95
nerve pain 155, 158
nervous system 30, 51, 68, 141, 198, 226-7
nettle rash 190
neurogenesis 8-9
nipple chafe 175-6
norethisterone 119-20
noses 49, 53-4, 63
NSAIDs (non-steroidal anti-inflammatories) 94-5, 97, 210-11
numbness in feet 152-3

obesity 113, 114, 115, 124, 154
otoconia 20
oesophagus 66, 69
oestrogen 97, 99, 104, 111, 218
oligomenorrhoea 122
optic neuritis 23
orgasms 100, 112, 114
orthotics, shoe 149
osteoarthritis 142, 143, 144-6
osteoporosis 122, 146-7, 149, 150, 218
ostomy bags and stomas 83
over-training/over-training syndrome 8, 122, 124, 204-5
overactive bladder (OAB) 103-4, 221
overactive thyroid/hyperthyroidism 34
oxygen distribution 28, 29, 33, 37, 39, 49, 50, 52, 53, 61-2

palpitations 28, 34-5, 43
paracetamol 26, 136, 148, 169, 210
paronychia 192-3
passive stretching 137
patella (knee cap) 143, 151
patellofemoral pain syndrome (PFPS) 151-2
peeing blood 96-7
pelvic floor muscles 89, 98-100, 101-2, 128, 132
   strengthening exercises 98, 99-101, 107, 128
pelvic stability 139, 151
penis, the 109, 110, 114, 186
perimenopause 130-1
periods, absent 121-2, 124, 218
periods, controlling 119-20
peripheral neuropathy 153
petroleum jelly 54
physiotherapists 149, 151, 157, 162, 163, 166, 168, 170, 208, 212
   women's health 98, 128, 129
piles 84-5
pins and needles 152-3
piriformis syndrome 164-5
placenta praevia 126
plantar fasciitis 154, 156-8
plasters/tape 176, 179

pollen 22, 54-5
pollution, air 64
polycystic ovary syndrome 122
polyps 63, 123
poo, blood in 77, 85
pooing/excretion 66, 74-7, 78, 79, 85, 99, 107, 128-9
post activation potentiation 226
post-natal depression 129
posture 4, 26, 64, 72, 142, 161, 167
pre-eclampsia 124, 126
pre-race nerves 74, 76, 78, 112
precooling 222
pregnancy 37, 97, 111, 122, 124-5, 126-7, 136
premature ejaculation 100
PRICE protocol 163, 209
productive running 12, 13-14
prolapsed discs 166
prolapses, vaginal 101-2, 128
prostaglandins 95
prostate, the 95, 96, 102-3, 104, 109-10
pulse 30, 34, 81

Radar keys 107
rashes, skin 185, 189-90
Raynaud's disease 36, 225
red blood cells 38, 39-40, 41, 125
RED-S (relative energy deficiency in sport) 218
reddening facial skin 196-7
relaxation techniques 220-1
renin/renin-angiotensin system 89
respiratory tract infections 203
reproductive system
   aching testicles 116-17
   anatomy of female 111-12
   anatomy of male 109-10
   checking your testicles 117, 132
   conceiving and running 124
   intermenstrual bleeding 123
   male fertility and sperm count 114-15
   menstrual cycle 118-22, 124, 132
   miscarriages 124, 125-6
   perimenopause 130-1
   pregnancy and running 126-7
   running after childbirth 128-9, 132
   sex and running 112-14
rescue breaths 45
resistance training 140, 144-5
respiratory system, anatomy of 49-51
rest days 214-15
resting heart rate 30
restless leg syndrome 137
retina detachment 23
rhabdomyolysis 97
rib cage 51
ring worm 185
rosacea 197
runner's high 6-7
runner's knee 151-2
runner's trots 74-7
runny nose/rhinitis 53-4

salbutamol 57, 58
salicylic acid 188
saliva 66, 68
salt levels, body 70, 89, 90, 91
salt water soaks 187-8

scarves 54, 55, 56, 197, 225–6
sciatic nerve 164, 165–6
sciatica 165–6
scrotum, the 109, 115, 116, 185
self-care 200–1
  eating disorders 218
  energy levels 219–20
  how much to run 227–8
  long-term medical conditions 205–6
  over-training 204–5
  recovery time and rest days 212, 214–15
  running and illness/recovery 201–4
  running and injuries 208–14, 229
  running in hot and cold weather 222–6
  sleep issues 220–1
  weight loss 216–17
sex and running 112–14
shin splints 147–9, 150
shoes, running 149, 152–3, 158, 160, 168,
  170, 179, 191, 193, 199
showers and bathing 21, 54, 106, 117, 136,
  174, 185, 186, 187, 195, 196, 199
sinusitis 63–4, 201
skin, anatomy of 172–4
  skin cancer 182
  skin infections 184–9
  skin, long-term conditions 194–8
  skin, protection 181–2
sleep 19, 26, 80, 115, 131, 204, 213, 220–1
slipped discs 166
slow-twitch fibres 137–8
smoking 11, 47, 64, 69, 132, 149, 177
snotty nose 53–4
socks 178, 179, 191, 193
sodium levels 91
sperm and semen 102, 109–10, 111,
  114–15, 116
spine, cervical 166–7
spit, need to 68
sports bras 174–5, 177
sports drinks 33, 71, 91, 130
sprained ankles 162–3
sprinting 63, 137, 138
squamous cell carcinoma (SCC) 182
static stretches 138, 139, 170
steroid injections 157, 158, 170
stitch 71–3
stomach, the 66, 69, 70, 85
Strassburg Socks 157, 158
strength and conditioning training 139–40,
  149, 170, 194, 214, 227–8, 229
stress 26, 34, 58, 59, 77–8, 85, 113, 115, 124,
  190, 204, 213, 220
stress fractures 150–1, 155
stress incontinence 97–8
stretching 72, 137, 138–9, 162, 164–5, 170, 227
strokes 23, 25, 28
subarachnoid haemorrhage (SAH) 25
subungual haematomas 191
Sudocrem 85
sunburn 182
sunglasses 22, 26, 54, 181, 222
sunscreen 181, 183, 199, 222
supplements, dietary 38–40, 41, 82, 96, 150
sweating 70, 90, 91, 107, 174, 187, 189, 195,
  196, 197–8
swelling injuries 211

swimmer's ear/otitis externa 21
synovial fluid 226

talking, running and 62
tears 21–2, 23
telomeres 221
temperature, body 60, 71, 93, 106, 137, 198,
  201, 222, 223–6
tempo pace runs 62
tendonitis 154, 161
tendons 134, 154, 156–7, 160, 161–2
testicles 109, 116–17, 132
testosterone 110, 111
threshold pace runs 62
thrush 185–6
thyroid disorders 136, 137, 153, 219
tibia, the 143, 148, 149, 167
time management 11–12
tinea cruris 185
toenails 191–3
torsion 117
tranexamic acid 121
transit time, food 85
tubules 89, 91, 93
type 2 diabetes 42, 94, 113, 114, 216, 228

ulcers, gastrointestinal 94
ultramarathons 39–40, 93, 94, 96–7
underactive thyroid/hypothyroidism 122,
  137, 153, 219
underwear 116, 121, 174–5, 177
urethra 95, 102, 105–6, 110
urinary incontinence 97–100, 102, 107, 128–9
urinary system, anatomy of 87–9
urinary tract infections (UTIs) 104, 106
urine samples, taking 105
urticaria 190
uterus 101, 111

vagina 101–2, 111, 186, 187
varicocele 116
varicose veins 36–7
vascular dementia 10, 11
verruca 188–9
vertigo 20
viral illnesses 20, 47, 56, 60, 63–4, 190, 201
vision, blurred 21–3
vital capacity 60
vitamin B12
vitamin D 149
VO2 max 61–2
vocal cord dysfunction (VCD) 58
volunteer work 16, 27
vomiting 70–1, 78, 79

warm-ups 56, 71, 72, 75, 126, 138, 170, 212,
  226–7, 229
watering eyes 21–2
weather conditions 26, 53, 55, 57, 63, 68, 97,
  107, 222–6, 229
weight, body 11, 42, 47, 64, 69, 80, 98, 99,
  102, 113, 114, 115, 122, 124, 132, 142,
  143–4, 148, 170, 194, 216–17
wheezing 57, 58, 60
white blood cells 200–1
wind 73–4, 83
windpipe/trachea 49, 50, 51